P9-DEW-796

HOW TO LOOK TEN YEARS YOUNGER

※※※

ALSO BY ADRIEN ARPEL
Adrien Arpel's 3-Week Crash Makeover/Shapeover Beauty Program

HOW TO LOOK TEN YEARS YOUNGER

ADRIEN ARPEL

WITH

RONNIE SUE EBENSTEIN

ILLUSTRATIONS BY
GAIL SCHNEIDER

WARNER BOOKS

A Warner Communications Company

Warner Books Edition

Copyright © 1980 by Adrienne Newman

All rights reserved. No part of this book may be reprinted without permission. For information address Rawson, Wade Publishers, Inc., 630 Third Avenue, New York, N.Y. 10017.

This Warner Books Edition is published by arrangement with Rawson, Wade Publishers, Inc.

Warner Books, Inc., 75 Rockefeller Plaza, New York, N.Y. 10019

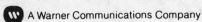 A Warner Communications Company

Printed in the United States of America

First Printing: May 1981

10 9 8 7 6 5 4 3 2 1

Color plates by Al Giese

Book design by Helen Barrow

Library of Congress Cataloging in Publication Data

Arpel, Adrien.
  How to look ten years younger.

  Includes index.
  1. Middle aged women—Health and hygiene.
2. Beauty, Personal. I. Ebenstein, Ronnie Sue,
joint author. II. Title.
RA778.A78   1981   613′.04244   80-21076
ISBN 0-446-97823-X (U.S.A.)
ISBN 0-446-97846-9 (Canada)

ATTENTION: SCHOOLS AND CORPORATIONS

WARNER books are available at quantity discounts with bulk purchase for educational, business, or sales promotional use. For information, please write to: SPECIAL SALES DEPARTMENT, WARNER BOOKS, 75 ROCKEFELLER PLAZA, NEW YORK, N.Y. 10019.

**ARE THERE WARNER BOOKS
YOU WANT BUT CANNOT FIND IN YOUR LOCAL STORES?**

You can get any WARNER BOOKS title in print. Simply send title and retail price, plus 50¢ per order and 50¢ per copy to cover mailing and handling costs for each book desired. New York State and California residents add applicable sales tax. Enclose check or money order only, no cash please, to: WARNER BOOKS, P.O. BOX 690, NEW YORK, N.Y. 10019. OR SEND FOR OUR COMPLETE CATALOGUE OF WARNER BOOKS.

To my beautiful sister, Marilyn

ACKNOWLEDGMENTS

I would like to thank John Kubie for his patience and support; all my friends in the field and offices of Seligman and Latz, Inc., with special thanks to Sunny Seitler; my dear friend Ronnie Sue Ebenstein, who is capable of writing successfully about anything with anyone; my publisher, Eleanor Rawson, for being terrific; Dr. Albert Shansky, a talented consulting chemist who, on his own time, served as my technical adviser for the formulas in this book; and all the doctors without whose help this book could never have been written. And I'd particularly like to thank Bill King for his outstanding cover photograph; Robert Anthony for his jacket design; Al Giese for all the fine book photography; Gail Schneider for her illustrating talent; and, most of all, those Arpel supervisors who made this book possible.

CONTENTS

❦❦❦

PART THREE

WELCOME TO MY STAY-YOUNG WORKSHOP

PART FOUR

HOW TO RECYCLE AND REDESIGN YOUR BODY VIA DIET, EXERCISE, AND CAMOUFLAGE

PART FIVE

HAIR: IT DOESN'T WRINKLE, BUT IT AGES

PART SIX

WHAT A DIFFERENCE A DAY MAKES

❦❦❦

A SPECIAL COLOR SECTION
FOLLOWS PAGE 194

PART ONE

✿✿✿

ARE YOU THE NEW IN-BETWEEN WOMAN?

CHAPTER 1

❦❦❦

The Subtract-10-Years System: Why You Should Start Today and What You Need to Know to Begin

I never put it into words before, but when I searched for a way to describe myself to you in the opening of this book, I began to wonder exactly how old I really am!

I have been performing beauty sleight of hand for so long (on myself as well as others) that I am no longer quite certain what belongs to me, what I've created, and how many years it took me to get from there to here.

OK, OK. Before you think I'm senile, I'll tell you: I'm close to 40—and in this book I promise to tell you how I learned to subtract 10 years from my looks and anyone else's in my work as head of my own cosmetics firm since the age of 17.

WELCOME TO THE TWILIGHT ZONE

I may be in my late 30s chronologically, but mentally and physically my age sort of hangs there in the "twilight zone." I'm not the same woman my mother was at this age, and neither, I'm sure, are you a stylized clone of your mother. For you and me, the new generation of over-25 women, chronological age can be, should be, irrelevant.

In the beginning, life was simple. If taking an age-related quiz in a Sunday supplement magazine, you would check one of the following boxes:

18–25, 26–45, 46+. And you (and I) would automatically be labeled by the box you checked:

18–25: young, sexy, feminine, working girl, student, dating.

26–45: wife and mother, staying dutifully at home, repeating that deadliest of phrases to your daughters, "When I was your age. . . ." Learning, flirting, working (and living) were supposed to slow down to a respectable energy-saving speed.

46+: mature, middle-aged, with one foot in the retirement generation, looking gleefully forward to spending evenings baby-sitting for grandchildren.

Well, the revolution in life styles that began in the 1960s has made these boxes inappropriate. If the 60s belonged to the society-changing "hippies" and the 70s ushered in the "therapy" generation, wherein "me" became the most important subject (reflected in best-selling titles like *Looking Out for Number One, Pulling Your Own Strings, How to Be Your Own Best Friend*), I don't need my crystal ball and tambourine to predict confidently that *the 80s will be the era of the new "in-between" woman*—the sexy, vital woman in her 30s and 40s+++ who still performs the many roles once reserved for younger "girls," from career woman to lover to mother, with the panache that comes with having experienced something of life—and, most important, with the looks of a woman 10 years younger than her driver's license claims. Looking forward to baby-sitting? We won't even have the time for sitting, baby!

WHO IS THE NEW IN-BETWEEN WOMAN?

There are millions of us out there who look, act, think, and feel younger than our birth certificates might indicate. We're not what the poets call the "young innocents," but we are interesting, experienced women who have learned how to effect an important "time freeze." While some women celebrate a birthday every year, or look as if they add a candle twice yearly, we manage to hold back the calendar till leap year rolls around. If you are ready for a more complex life style that demands a young-looking appearance, and you're ready to put into practice the stay-young system you're about to learn, you're ready to join our ranks.

And your age is irrelevant. You can be 40 and feel the need for a change, or you can be 25 years old, encased in a no-look "matronly" image, lacking young style and pizzazz. Either way, you need to learn how to project the physical image that goes with the mental picture you have of yourself. How can you transform your fantasized self-image into a new, younger beauty reality? You could time-travel to Camelot to make an appointment with Merlin the Magician (though I hear he's booked solid through 2001), but there is real beauty and health wizardry taking place closer to home, and you'll find it in this working manual geared for both young women in their 20s who are clever enough to take charge of their looks now, and for women like me (in their 30s/40s+++) who want to learn how to subtract 10 years from every part of their anatomy.

Consider this scenario: You're reading a magazine or watching TV and someone in the public eye comes into view. You know she's about your age, yet she looks so much younger, so "together." No, she doesn't have her own picture of Dorian Gray that she secretly allows to age in her stead. *She does have me and my team of experts—or someone like me—guiding her every beauty, health, and fashion step. And until now, you didn't.* If you were privy to the stay-young secrets she receives, you would also look younger, and terrific.

I've written this book to help you step into the above scenario, because I believe it is time to give you the results-producing routines that will keep your birthdays from showing up on your face and body, so you can have a head (and body) start on your new life style. You're about to close the 10-years-off information gap and join the clever in-between women who are willing to invest a little time and effort in their own dividend-paying beauty futures.

IMPORTANT POINT #1

You can't help being 29/36/43, but you can help looking like the last generation's idea of the over-25 woman. If someone can guess your age, you're not doing enough. *Why this book should be read by young women:* What you do to and for yourself in your mid-20s and 30s—the stay-young processes you follow—will determine how you will look in your 40s and beyond. *Why you need this book if you're an in-between woman:* You've already waved good-bye to 35? Don't feel you've passed the point of no return and curl up with a pint of strawberry sherbet or Stolichnaya vodka for solace. You can learn how to correct the mistakes you made in your formative years, so there's no excuse for not starting to read—and act—now.

TROMPE L'OEIL

The French have an expression for one of the important "how-tos" you'll learn in this book—*trompe l'oeil*, or, in English, "trick the eye." When you pass the age of consent, you have to learn the tricks taught to every jet setter, female politician, film personality—anyone who has stayed on top for years: the art of looking younger. And make no mistake, it is a *studied* art. Though it isn't publicized as openly as the Hollywood divorce-go-round, the women in front of the lens, for example, memorize camouflage tricks with even more ardor than they devote to the study of their lines. They learn from the experts the best ways to disguise a slightly thickening waist, how to emphasize the eyes and lips with make-up so no one notices a few lines, how to "tape" a slightly sagging breast to give a youthful bustline.

Think about it. You just don't see a beginning-to-age glamour symbol in a bikini; what you do see is a perfectly pulled-together woman who always looks so right you naturally assume she, unlike you, could carry off a tiny little two-piece perfectly. She can't, but no one notices. Because she still has smooth-looking, supple skin, a gloriously full head of hair, a slender (notice I didn't say perfect) body that she camouflages to *appear* perfect.

Why is she so blessed with ever-young physical attributes? The only difference between you and her is *education*. She has an MBA, Master of Beauty Arts. She also has access to highly qualified, high-priced teams of beauty experts: Her "professors" are talented doctors, make-up artists, hair designers, fashion coordinators, and more who, for a not inconsiderable sum, gladly whisper in her diamond-studded ears the suggestions that allow her to take 10 years off her face and every part of her body. Well, I've cornered these same experts, and in this book I've brought out into the open, out of the closet, the very beauty programs rich and successful women live by. I've also added the many subtract-a-year do-it-yourself tricks that have helped me, including:

- how to take 10 years off your looks in 10 minutes via correct make-up application
- how to take 10 years off your skin with fabulous Prescription Sleep Serums
- how to remove the wrinkles you do unto yourself with the Arpel Acupressure Adaptation
- how to avoid the over-30 matronly hairstyle syndrome
- how to lose 2 to 5 pounds in 24 hours
- how to choose mistake-proof hair color

- □ how to change your body shape by changing your underwear
- □ how to merchandise yourself into a class act by choosing the right (not necessarily most expensive) clothes . . . with a fashion co-ordinator's eye for stay-young styling

If you want to whisper the question, "How can I look ten years younger?" I've made the answers loud and clear.

"WELCOME TO THE MARKETPLACE" SEMINAR

Just how did I come to the conclusion that I wasn't the only woman who felt the need—and desire—to look 10 years younger? *You told me!*

As head of an international cosmetics company with 450 salons in major department stores all over the world, I travel a great deal (I've probably logged more fly-time than the most veteran of airline pilots), holding beauty and success seminars attended mostly by women in their mid to upper 20s to 40s, the new in-between women. Whether I'm at Saks Fifth Avenue in New York, Neiman-Marcus in Dallas, Macy's San Francisco, or Harrods of London, I've noticed that the accent may be different, but the one question sure to come up is: *How can I look younger?*

I've also noticed that both the reasons for and specifics of the question have changed greatly during the past ten years. While in the primordial early 60s I was often asked, "How can I look like Elizabeth Taylor or Brigitte Bardot?" today's woman has realistic goals in mind to match her need to stay young looking. Her main reason: *a change of life style, not change of life.*

Women are now entering all sorts of marketplaces, often for the first time, and they know they must create a new image to match their new reality. Witness:

- □ the divorced-and-suddenly-dating marketplace
- □ the kids-left-home, bored-with-the-empty-nest, back-to-work marketplace
- □ the PhD-in-business, how-do-I-look-feminine-yet-competent marketplace
- □ the 27-and-changing-to-a-glamour-career marketplace
- □ the 32-and-promoted-to-bank-VP marketplace
- □ the just-because-I'm-happy-at-home-doesn't-mean-I-want-to-be-out-of-it marketplace.

One thing all of these very different women agree on: This is a new world and it's here to stay, but whatever sphere you're planning to enter, whatever life change you're thinking of making, make no mistake, a young-looking, well-put-together look will make you more comfortable and confident while you're trying to achieve your goal. Yes, it would be wonderful if our brains, talent, and selfless personalities alone could help us get what we want, but reality just doesn't make it so. If two Harvard Business School graduates were equally qualified candidates for the same job, I assure you that the one who looked right, who created the successful, young, and important image would get the position. An employer, for example, is not just buying your brains—she/he is interested in the total package you present.

That is why if I give one warning at a seminar, it is this: *Don't be a shelf flower* (the packaging version of a wallflower, a product that's languishing on the shelf). Everyone who wants to make a major life change, or improve her current situation, should consider herself a product looking to enhance her share of the market. And if you aren't "selling" well (aren't achieving what you set out to accomplish), you need to learn new techniques to get your image across, to stand out from all the other "packages" on the shelf. You must ask yourself, "What's wrong with this package?" and learn how to give yourself the edge that can help turn you from a no sale/low sale product into a success story.

Don't get me wrong: I am not a psychiatrist, marriage counselor, or executive recruiter. But I am a beauty executive who knows that looking young (not 18 years old; I'm not a genie and this is no fairy tale!) and well put together can help you get where you want to go. That's why I stress a system that shows how to stave off the first signs of aging, remove some "over-21" signs that have already appeared, and, equally important, how to camouflage what can't be changed. It's a system that revamps your total package—not just your skin or hair.

How did this system develop? Out of my need to answer fully the new questions asked by the new in-between woman who was interested in keeping premature aging at bay rather than just looking "pretty-pretty." To complete my research portfolio re *ease-on aging*, i.e., sliding from one birthday to the next with a barely noticeable change in appearance, I asked doctors and beauty professionals the questions you were asking me, including:

- □ What kind of night creams and treatment products will help my suddenly tending-to-dry skin . . . still-breaking-out skin . . . accordion-pleated, wrinkled skin?
- □ How do I use make-up to hide the negatives like incipient laugh lines . . . starting-to-crinkle eyelids?
- □ I'm thin, but after two babies/my 30th birthday (pick one), I've developed a pot belly. How can I flatten my stomach?

- When I wear a low-cut dress, it looks as though my breasts are low-cut, too. What kind of bra will give me natural-looking cleavage?
- I've exercised off what I can. How do I camouflage these spreading hips?
- What can I do for lining skin . . . thinning hair . . . crow's-feet . . . less-than-firm thighs?
- I'd rather be a Ferrari than a Ford: How can I look like a status package on a brand-X budget?

This book, then, is the result of the anti-aging notebooks I've kept for my beauty seminars and store appearances. It also grew out of the important information I couldn't fit into my first book, *Adrien Arpel's 3-Week Crash Makeover/Shapeover Beauty Program*, in which I attempted to answer many of the beauty and health questions women frequently asked me. But there was *so much* that could be done to help a woman look younger longer, I couldn't answer the years-off questions in a few paragraphs or even a chapter. When I found the anti-aging questions were taking up much of the seminar sessions, I realized the system I had put together warranted the full treatment, a book of its own. I truly am convinced you can look 10 years younger than you are chronologically, and I'm willing to talk openly and out loud about exactly what it takes to do so.

And I promise you, the system you'll follow will be realistic. True, a month at a Swiss sleep clinic might put your weight problem, to say nothing of your insomnia, to rest—but I doubt if a lengthy dissertation on what to pack for such a "coma cure" will help smooth away one wrinkle or help you shed one pound. When I decided I wanted to look 10 years younger, I knew that I, as a working woman, wife, and mother, didn't have one minute to waste with beauty fluff and nonsense—and I'm sure you don't either. So I've put together a working manual that works . . . if you'll work with it.

I also must confess I wanted this book to make sense for personal reasons. My first book was a national best seller, and the feedback I've received from readers who recommended it to their friends tells me it was successful because it was realistic and the advice worked. I want this stay-young system to do the same.

IMPORTANT POINT #2

If you're like me, you don't have hours to spend basting yourself with a preservative and staring (or swearing!) at your mirrored reflection. Nor do you have the time to sit around dreaming about returning to those golden days of yesteryear. That's why this book is filled with *short-cuts*, time-saving tips, things to do (and not do) that will give you maximum results in a minimum amount of time. But you do have to devote some thought and effort to what you'll be reading and doing. There is no miracle housed in these pages; you won't look 10 years younger simply by wishing it were so.

NO EXCUSES

Of course, the process of aging can't be stopped (if I could accomplish that feat, I'd be lecturing at the Mayo Clinic instead of at Saks), but it can be slowed, not just by your best friend, but by you. I hear all sorts of reasons women give for why someone *else* looks younger:

- She's small-boned, so she's maintained her figure.
- She's artistic, so she applies make-up well.
- She's always been athletic, so she's never too tired to exercise.

Well, your young-looking friend doesn't owe her looks to her astrological sign or biorhythm chart. She works at it, and she's realistic enough to have started her 10-years-off routines at an age when most women still find laugh lines funny.

@#$%¢! = AGING

You can join her, and the other in-between women who will look terrific long after they can no longer be mistaken for ingénues, by changing your attitude toward that dirtiest of words, aging. First, admit that it will happen. From 25 on, you'll notice subtle changes taking place . . . on your best friend, if not on yourself. (At your high school reunions, you'll think everyone looks older but you.) Young girls in their early 20s often come to me and say, "It seems like I have crow's-feet/laugh lines/drying, flaky skin. It's not possible, is it?" Well, I hate to tell you: If it's there, it's possible, but it certainly isn't the beginning of the end. There's so much that can be done to keep signs of premature aging from getting the upper hand, why not start now?

Scientists tell us that chronologically everyone ages at more or less the same rate, give or take a few years. *But everyone doesn't look the same at the same age.* The sooner you learn to change the habits that add totally unnecessary years to your looks, the more successfully you'll beat the age trap. There are hundreds of ways to slow the aging process, and I've catalogued them for you in this book.

To fight aging successfully (whether you want to look 10 years younger than your chronological age or to look like a "together" 25-year-old rather than a blah 25-going-on-who-cares), you must understand the subtle changes taking place daily on your face and within your body. You need to know how and why a wrinkle forms to keep it from happening. You must understand dehydration of the skin in order to stop it. You must be prepared to work off those body flaws that can be eliminated. And you must be realistic about body changes that appear as early as your mid-20s, changes that stubbornly refuse to go away. You accept them, and you learn how to camouflage cleverly to show the best and hide the worst. *But learning is just the beginning, because knowledge is useless without a system of action.* This book will provide you with the detailed beauty and health system that will make you look 10 years younger: You're now holding in your hands a complete Stay-Young Workshop.

LIFE, EUROPEAN-STYLE

Our sisters across the sea have really written the first chapter of any stay-young guide. In Europe an 18-year-old may be considered a thing of beauty, but she wouldn't keep a man rapt with joy forever. That's because the European good-looks ideal is different from ours, and a common fantasy on this side of the Atlantic is often played out in real life "over there": In any café in the most romantic foreign city, you will often see a young, virile-looking man staring with undivided attention at his feminine, very attractive (yet decidedly over-30) companion.

This woman looks right, not ridiculous, sipping a vermouth cassis with a younger man because she's combined the sophistication and experience of a woman her age *with the face and body of a woman 10 years her junior.* She makes the winsome, obviously inexperienced young girls at the next table look light-years away, on a lower planet.

In the United States we're just beginning to take this European ideal of sophisticated beauty seriously. When *Harper's Bazaar* named America's 10 great beauties in their April 1978 issue, quite a stir was raised when it was noted the chosen were all over age 30—a few of them hadn't seen 40 in a while. But they did all look sensual and healthy, relaxed and confident, with smooth skin, thick hair, and all the trappings we associate with young women.

They projected fabulous good looks because they have been *trained* in the art of taking care of themselves—the same multifaceted art you'll learn in the chapters that follow.

IMPORTANT POINT #3

The women who awe us—who are so attractive and confident, who have the best jobs, the glamour careers and life styles—are *not* picture-perfect, delicately featured visions of Elizabethan beauty still too young to vote. They are the older sisters and mothers of these girls, who combine exciting good looks with the sophistication that only comes with putting some distance between themselves and their 21st birthdays. Remember, if your general appearance and the "vibes" you give out are young and good looking, that is all anyone will ever see.

PART TWO

HOW TO GET FROM 25 TO INFINITY PRACTICALLY WRINKLE-FREE

CHAPTER 2

❦❦❦

The Big-Six Skin Battle Zones: How to Beat the Premature Agers

If you can greet your first wrinkle with a squeal of delight and consider a furrowed brow a badge of graceful maturity, you're either browbeaten or uncommonly unvain. And you're definitely in the minority. Most of the women I meet on my promotional beauty tours are about as willing to usher in signs of facial aging as they would be to open their doors, smiling, to their husbands' younger second wives.

I certainly fall into the latter group, the I'd-rather-fight-than-wrinkle majority. And since I feel growing old gracefully should be left to those who were never gracefully *young*, I cajoled and persuaded the doctors and other beauty professionals who work to keep skin young looking to share their secrets and techniques with me.

My most important discovery: If you know how to fight (and beat) the *Bix-Six Skin Battles*, you can win the war on aging and keep your skin looking at least 10 years younger than it really is chronologically. So roll up your sleeves (I'll discuss upper arm problems later) and start reading.

While tradition has it that pride goeth before a fall, ignorance—and gravity—goeth before the fall of your epidermis. The six most important reasons your skin looks 10 years older than it has to are: 1) Internal Dermal Happenings, 2) Heredity, 3) Environment, 4) Bad Habits, 5) Remembrance of Skin Problems Past, 6) Signs of Time. The means to fight these six skin battles and a host of other premature agers are discussed in the pages that follow. But in order to know how to save your skin, to keep its youth-retaining powers in perpetual motion, you first have to understand how skin works, what keeps it young looking . . . and what doesn't.

The decline and fall of the epidermis begins at around age 25 and leads to Tactical Skin Error #1: waiting too long before beginning an informed skin-care ritual. Remember, when it comes to saving face, *it is easier to deter than bring back*. So, to those of you who are reading this at age 25, bravo! You're here at the right time. You're past 25 and fear the only way to bring your skin back to life is via a séance with your legendary great-grandmother who died with perfect skin at 98? Now that it's later in the game for your skin, you'll have to be more diligent (forget magic—your séance might conjure up the genes from the bad-skinned side of the family!); I'll give you the techniques to revive and repair your skin in this and the following four chapters.

You're younger than 25? Even better. I see this book as a sweet-16 gift —not a menopause guide! I meet so many young women who are lined and needn't be—and it need not happen to you.

Here, in brief, is what happens: Skin, as your high school hygiene teacher probably told you, is divided into two layers, the epidermis and the dermis. The epidermis is the outer layer. It serves to protect your skin from the hazards of the environment and to make sure that the rest of you doesn't ooze out and blow away. The lower layers of the epidermis are really a beehive of activity. This is where young cells are constantly being formed. The young cells mature, make their way to the surface of the epidermis, and die. By the time they reach the top, they're actually completely dead, made up of a hard, horny substance called *keratinized protein*. "KP" needs water to look supple and feel youthful—lack of water near the skin's surface causes the keratin to become brittle and your skin to look and feel dry, whether you're 20 or 60. Luckily for us, the top dead layer is sloughed off continuously and replaced with young, healthy cells from beneath the surface. (As we tearfully say goodbye to our 20s, it becomes vital to speed up this sloughing process—more about this later.)

While the no-longer-18 epidermis gives rise to that mirror sadness known as "what you see is what you get," the true perpetrators of lines, bags, sags, and wrinkles lie in the invisible-to-us dermis, comfortably nestled out of the limelight, just beneath the epidermis. The dermis forms the support system of the skin. It is the home of oil and sweat glands, hair follicles, blood vessels, and fat glands. It also houses collagen, that all-important elastic protein that keeps your skin young, malleable, and supple.

Now that you know what your skin is made of, let's get to the nitty-gritty. Rather than give you a lecture on skin transformations, I've put the necessary information in the form of Questions and Answers, so you can relate changes in the form and function of skin to the changes you see in your mirror. I've also prescribed some treatments to do now to keep you looking terrific later; these "prescriptions" are listed in ℞ form along with the answers to many of the questions.

INTERNAL DERMAL HAPPENINGS

You mention that a lot goes on inside the dermis, the skin's inner layers, that affects our skin's appearance. . . . What actually happens, and can we control it?

Several physiological happenings contribute to skin changes—changes that can make you look older prematurely.

Collagen Collapse

This is a biggie! Collagen (and elastin, another protein) is the fibrous connective tissue that physically supports your face. From the moment you leave the shelter of the womb, your collagen starts to age and decrease in amount, and new collagen is no longer produced in copious quantities as you get older. There's also something called "cross-linkage" taking place: The collagen fibers keep on intertwining until they form a hard mass rather than a series of nicely malleable strands. While this tightening collagen helps turn your baby fat into firm 19-year-old flesh, the *continued* cross-linking that goes on forever gives you less resilient skin and you lose the bounce-back factor, which works like this: When you smile, groan, or yawn, elastic collagen helps the skin bounce back to its normal position following a change of expression. When there is less elasticity, temporary expression lines and wrinkles become permanent, your skin actually becomes too big for the impaired network of collagen and fat that supports it, and it starts to bag and sag.

To counteract collagen collapse, there are a few simple steps you can take right now.

℞. *Decrease sun exposure.* The sun viciously attacks collagen, turning your skin into peanut brittle in the process.

℞. *Wear a day cream* that contains collagen protein to boost your own supply. It will be listed on the label as collagen or hydrolized animal protein.

℞. *Increase your vitamin C intake.* C produces collagen; your body can't produce and store enough of this beauty vitamin to help your skin make it through the years without help. A 100-mg supplement daily is in order; so is a diet rich in citrus fruits.

Desiccation and Water Loss

As a result of these two dermis-related wrinkle disasters, your skin literally dries up and the outer layer gets flaky as the acid mantle winds down over the years. This acid mantle you hear so much about is composed of oil from the sebaceous glands, old-fashioned sweat, and other valuable secretions, which sit on top of the epidermis, bathing the skin in a protective coating that helps prevent the skin's own moisture (i.e., water) from evaporating and helps keep environmental enemies like wind and pollution at bay. As the 25+ skin ages, the sebum- and sweat-producing glands wither, so important fluids can't get to the surface in great enough quantity to protect your skin. Result: You actually lose water content because of a faulty acid mantle and a cracked epidermis!

℞. *The solution: rehydration* . . . a not-so-technical term meaning replacement of lost water. And because we're saying moisture content is related to water, not oil or grease, oily-skinned women need to rehydrate as conscientiously as their dry-skinned sisters, and then add the right kind of moisturizer to compensate for their defective acid mantle.

You will rehydrate externally if you leave your skin damp after you wash your face, then lock in the water film by applying moisturizer. Whenever you can, spray water on your face and reapply moisturizer.

You can also replace lost skin-cell water internally by drinking six to eight glasses of water a day. The ancient Egyptians made a big mistake. Instead of praying to the sun god, they should have knelt on their knees and done incantations along the banks of the Nile. Because the greatest youth—giving/keeping food/drink is water.

Sluggish Circulation

Among other things, the dermis contains the blood vessels, which are conductors of nourishment and eliminators of waste. When the intracellular blood flow slows down, so does the creation of new cellular matter. The blood doesn't get a chance to flow close enough to the surface to let a pink, healthy glow radiate through.

℞. *Stimulate the circulation.* While you can't control blood flow, you can *stimulate* it—with exercises that work facial muscles. I'll clue you in with the special Arpel Acupressure Adaptation, described in Chapter 5. You can also *simulate* the rosy glow good circulation provides by doing the following:

℞. *Help the blood flow reach the face via a slantboard*—any well-padded board about six feet long upon which you lie on your back with your feet angled two feet higher than your head, with your head near the floor. Prop the foot of the board securely against a chair that won't skid. Ten minutes, three times daily, on a slantboard moves the blood up to your face, takes a load off your legs and that blood-moving muscle, your heart. . . . It's also a terrific energizer.

℞. *Slough the skin regularly* to remove the dead, gray-looking top layer of your epidermis. If you understand what skin sloughing or epidermabrasion does, you'll understand why it should be part of your beauty routine, so I want to explain the procedure in some detail.

As I mentioned earlier, by the time your skin's cell factory pushes new, young cells up through the several layers of epidermis to the surface, these cells are dead, and the longer they lie on top of your skin and accumulate, the longer they block younger cells from coming up to take their place and replenish your face. These oldies are not goodies. They're really just hanging around accumulating cellular debris and waste, making your skin look dull and muddy, forming an invisible grayish skin callus. You remove this "callus" by sloughing/epidermabrading/exfoliating (same thing) . . . and help restore your skin's lively, youthful glow. (Too bad we can't rejuvenate the rest of our bodies this easily!)

While the acne sufferer benefits because sloughing helps unplug the blocked pore openings filled with the excess oil that forms blackheads, the rest of us benefit by speeding up the march of healthy young cells to the skin's surface.

Sloughing Materials

There are a variety of sloughing tools on the market, both mechanical and cosmetic. In the mechanical area, there are complexion brushes that you can work over your skin to exfoliate—just make sure your brush, whether battery-powered or hand-held, has natural bristles. Or you might want to try 3M's Buf-Puf, a dermatologist-designed synthetic sponge that's strictly for exfoliating. (Note: You don't exfoliate without cleanser—you work the brush into your chosen soap/cleanser first, *then* work it over wet, lathered skin.)

You can also use your fingertips, along with gritty cleansers that are sold at cosmetic counters. These special cleansers combine mild abrasives (i.e., almonds, corn meal, oatmeal) with skin soothers (various oils, honey) in a cream base. When you remove the massaged-in abrasive cleanser, you remove some of the cellular debris along with it.

There's another slightly more exotic exfoliant—the at-home commercial peels made by many cosmetic companies. They, too, will help you peel away the top, dead layer, leaving younger-looking skin behind.

You've learned the face-sloughing *whats* and *whys* (I'll teach you *how often* in the next chapter).

℞. *Seasonal slough tip.* Your skin's cell factory works overtime in warm weather, speeding up cell production and shedding. Adjust your summer skin-care schedule to include more frequent sloughing to match your skin's suddenly upbeat tempo.

℞. *Slough your body*—especially where dead skin tends to accumulate (elbows, knees, feet). A natural sea sponge or a luffa works well on the body, but keep it in the bath; it's too rough for facial skin.

Three ℞s *for the bath:*

▫ Slather on oil before you enter the tub (natural sesame oil is an excellent skin softener), lotion when you step out.

▫ Don't wash with overly hot water. It strips oil from the skin.

▫ Don't loll in the tub forever (especially in winter when your skin is drier to begin with); you run the risk of overhydrating your skin. The cells may become swollen with water, giving you that puckered-prune effect.

HEREDITY . . .

When I look at my favorite family photo, I'm glad I inherited my mother's and grandmother's blonde hair. But now that my face is starting to crinkle . . . I wonder if I'll also wind up with their accordion-pleated skin?

Unfortunately, heredity does play a large part in the who-wrinkles-when lottery. Your family's skin-type tree will tell you a lot about what you can expect to happen to your own skin in the future. Black skin stays young looking longer because it has more pigment to protect collagen from the sun's damaging ultraviolet rays. If your ancestors hail from the Mediterranean or the Middle East, you will no doubt have a thicker, oilier skin that won't wrinkle as fast as the skin of fair-haired women of Nordic descent. If you have what the dermatologists call "Celtic coloring"—blue eyes and red hair

—your skin is probably thin, too. Skin thickness varies—and thin skin wrinkles faster.

Of course, few of us are solely one skin type. Our roots are diverse, and that's why everyone's skin changes at a slightly different rate. But you can look to your parents and to both sets of grandparents for a clue as to what might happen.

Does that mean you're doomed to repeat your mother's wrinkle pattern crease for crease, sag for sag? Fortunately, no. Once you understand your genetic tendencies, you can improve your skin—via the proper treatment regimens, which I will teach you. You can't change your roots, but you can help alter your skin's destiny by improving its environment.

. . . vs. ENVIRONMENT

I seem to look 5 years younger, and much healthier, with a tan. The sun is supposed to be the source of life. . . . Isn't all its bad press exaggerated?

Would you believe that most, if not all, dermatologists say sun exposure is the *number 1* cause of aging? Some M.D.'s go even further, believing that chronological age has *nothing whatsoever* to do with aging skin . . . that a 40-year-old woman who was never exposed to sun would have smooth, youthful-looking skin, while a nubile California surfer type who's out catching the rays several hours a day can have the face of an old crone.

Whether or not sun is the only factor, the scientific community is in major agreement on one point: It's the greatest factor in *premature* aging, because the sun is a prime collagen destroyer, making the skin dry out and harden, which can lead to a condition called keratosis, a precursor of skin cancer. The sun destroys collagen by passing through the epidermis (which thins as you get older anyway) and attacking the collagen nestled in the dermal tissues. Just study your skin where it's *not* exposed to the sun: the buttocks, under your breasts, inside your forearm . . . your entire skin would look that smooth throughout middle age if you lived underground.

But before you decide to burrow, understand that skin pigmentation, too, affects how each person will react to sunlight. The blue-eyed redhead will burn eight times as fast as the black woman. In fact, Australia has the world's highest rate of skin cancer because it is the only country where Caucasians live so close to the equator. One dermatological wag asks, "What do you call white people who live in the sun?" The answer: "Patients."

And the doctor is right: Where you live can make you look 10 years older than you really are. I see the evidence in my own business travels. If women who live in Arizona, Hawaii, Florida, and other hot spots are not very careful, they may tend to look older than Eastern seaboard inhabitants. I used to envy them the fabulous weather in the sunbelt; now I know that when the Lord giveth he also taketh away! You don't have to *lie* in the sun to experience these ill effects—if you're not careful, you just have to *live* in a sunny clime to get that slightly weather-beaten look.

The sun is no respecter of wealth, as I demonstrated in a story for a newspaper published in a sun-drenched city. We took a fabulously wealthy woman who had spent her whole life outdoors (sailing, sunning, golfing) and a migrant farm woman of the same age who also was an "outdoors-woman" (she spent brutal days picking crops under the burning sun) and covered both their heads with turbans. And do you know, you couldn't tell which was which—the pampered millionairess looked as prematurely aged as the migrant farm worker. The moral of this little tale is obvious, so I won't repeat it.

Another unfortunate fact about the sun: Its damage is progressive—those ultraviolet rays you received from last summer's sunburn are still working to destroy your skin this winter. So the sooner you stop sunning yourself (even if you're careful never to burn), the better off your skin will be. While hibernation and total avoidance will work, more practical sun-repelling steps exist. Southern women a few generations back used parasols—for good reason. Today, whether you're from Birmingham, Alabama, or Binghamton, New York, if you are wise, when the sun shines you will wear a brimmed hat . . . and take the following anti-sun precautions.

℞. *Sunscreens.* Look for one containing proven burn fighters, either 5 percent PABA (like PreSun or Eclipse) or benzophenone (found in Uval, Solbar) and reapply it often. If you can't avoid spending a great deal of time in the sun, mix your screens—alternate application of both types so you'll get double the chemical protection. If you're a downhill racer or cross-country skier, try RVP. It protects against high-altitude windburns, too.

℞. *Sunblocks.* To block out physically as many UV-B rays (they're the ultraviolets that do the most destruction), use a sunblock containing zinc oxide or titanium dioxide.

Dot your block over the screen in areas of greatest exposure: nose, cheekbones, lips, etc. Better to look as though you're auditioning for Ringling Bros. for a few hours than to live with a burn, peeling, and other unpleasantness for days (not to mention hidelike skin years later).

℞. *Take action—take aspirin.* You've already sinned and overdone the sun? Dr. Robert Auerbach, associate professor of clinical dermatology at New York University Medical Center, New York City, suggests you can help yourself if you act *before* your skin starts to redden by taking two aspirins. Besides having analgesic (pain-deadening) ability, aspirin helps prevent ultraviolet damage by slowing down your skin's inflammation-producing mechanism. (Exception: If you're dehydrated, skip the aspirin. Instead, drink plenty of cold water and prepare for your burning punishment.)

℞. *Steam.* If you have oily skin that you find encapsulated by a thick crust of tan, give your face an herbal steam bath. Put 2 tablespoons of herbs (camomile or rosemary is nice) into a large pot of boiling water. Remove pot from stove, make a tent by draping a towel over both the pot and your head, and steam for 5 minutes, making sure you keep face 6 inches from pot. (Note: If you have normal to dry skin, steaming isn't for you. Moisturize instead.)

Sun Spots

Wrinkles and the leathery look aren't the only legacy of sun worshiping. You can also develop uneven (unattractive) brown patches on your face, chest, arms, and hands known as liver spots, and—surprise—age has nothing to do with the condition. If you've spent summers hanging out in the sun since you were 15, you could have these hyperpigmented "senile freckles" at the age of 30. (The only time you get sun is when you're skiing in the winter? If you don't wear a sunscreen, you're getting supreme sun damage. Snow reflects 85 percent of the ultraviolet rays. Instead, try spending your outdoor spare time exercising on the grass, which reflects only 2.5 percent of the harmful rays.)

If you have these spots, you've done permanent damage to the mottled areas, and senile freckles can't be rejuvenated. They can, however, be removed in many cases. The magical spot remover is no magician, he's your skilled dermatologist, who may use one of three methods: 1) cryosurgery—a freezing process; 2) electrosurgery—employment of a needle propelled by electricity (also called electrodesiccation); or 3) chemosurgery—a chemical peel making use of acids.

You have to do your part. Stay out of the sun or wear a good skin-protecting agent. You've read about those Caribbean vacation clubs where an add-a-bead necklace pays for extra drinks, etc. I call them add-a-year clubs!

Now that I've done permanent damage to the sun's reputation, I'd like to continue my environmental attack with a few nasty words about other youth robbers.

Gone with the . . .

A windburn is to be avoided. Not only does it aim destructively for your epidermis, giving you that cracked, dry feeling . . . it also robs you of the moisture nestled in your dermis, giving you premature dry skin wrinkles.

℞. *Going out on a windy day?* Wear a nourishing day cream containing lanolin, a rich emollient derived from the sebaceous glands of a sheep, as well as your moisturizer to seal your own moisture in and keep the wind from drying you out.

The Big "P"

Pollution eats away at your skin (The sulfur dioxide in the air gnaws at granite buildings; what makes you think your face is immune?) and gives your complexion a grayish/yellowish cast that's far from the rosy glow of youth.

℞. *Slough off the dead, pollution-coated top layer* of skin, or have a professional facial weekly if you live in a big city with poor air quality.

Heat Wave

Just when you thought it was safe to stay indoors . . . you have to worry about the effects of central heating on your skin. The problem is this: Your skin's softness is in direct proportion to its water content, which is held in the skin by the protective acid mantle. As you pass the first-time voter age by 5 years or so, outer layers of your skin become thinner, as noted. The oily acid mantle isn't as oily as it used to be . . . so the water leaches out into the environment. Now, if the environment is dry, because of central heating or air conditioning, it will rob your skin of its moisture more rapidly. To counteract dry rooms, which can be more beauty-destroying than dry rot:

℞. *Get a humidifier.* It's a greater dividend-producing investment than a face-lift. Rather than have your skin donate its limited moisture content to the air while you sleep (this is one kind of charity that *shouldn't* begin at home), let your pores inhale the humidifier's output. A room with a high moisture content is what you're aiming for. How to tell? Your plants won't shrivel, your throat won't feel dry when you wake up.

℞. *Surround yourself with greenery.* Plants add moisture to the air . . . which your skin will thirstily absorb.

℞. *Turn the thermostat as far down as possible* when you sleep. One reason clever European women look young so much longer than many of us is that they know cold is a preservative. If you turn your thermostat down to 62 degrees before bedtime and pile on the blankets the way frugal Europeans do, you'll be helping preserve your skin's youthful state. After all, they keep meat fresh and furs young looking by putting them in cold storage; why not do the same for your face?

The Plane Truth

There's yet another environmental hazard you may not be aware of, and that's the effect of air travel on your skin. The compression in the cabin, combined with the ever-present air conditioning, is very drying. If you're a frequent air traveler, you need some in-flight training. Instead of drinking the cocktails offered by the stewards, drink plenty of mineral water. (I'm waiting for the day the airline attendants will say, "Coffee, tea, or Perrier?") Here are three prescriptions for plane travel:

R. *At the start of the trip*, drink three-quarters of a bottle of mineral water and pat the rest onto your skin with a cotton ball (keep in a plastic bag for just this purpose); repeat at intervals. On the trip from New York to LA, for example, I drink at least four glasses of mineral water and pat a cupful on my face.

R. *Apply moisturizer before boarding*, and reapply frequently.

R. *Keep your eye oil handy*, and use it liberally between takeoff and landing.

By doing the above you can turn the getting-there portion of any flight into a several-hour moisture-replenishing treatment, something you don't have the time or inclination for on land. It will also give you something to think about besides the state of the landing gear and the skill of the pilot!

BAD HABITS

There are certain vices I find hard to give up—notably cigarettes and alcohol. Will these habits make my skin look older?

While scientists debate among themselves the whys of the smoking-wrinkles relationship, they are in agreement that smoking definitely does prematurely age the skin, especially around the eyes and upper lip. The deeper, earlier crow's-feet of smokers could be due to the fact that for each cigarette you smoke, your body is depleted of about 25 mg of vitamin C, and, as I mentioned earlier, C is important to collagen production. Eye-area collagen decay could also be caused by the squinting that's a natural defense against smoke wafting up toward your eyes. Cigarettes can also contribute to wrinkling around the mouth, for purely mechanical reasons. Next time you light up, observe how your mouth scrunches up whenever you take a puff. . . . Smoking is *not* a recommended facial exercise. While you may be aware of nicotine-stained fingertips, you may *not* realize that smoking can also make your skin look sallow—some researchers think that smoking impairs blood circulation.

As for alcohol, you can be sure that the French person who said, "A day without wine is like a day without sunshine," would have changed his motto if he realized those luscious grapes turn to dried-up raisins! Alcohol, like sun, is aging. So if you don't want to wither on the vine, you'd better moderate your daily dose of the grape. While an occasional drink won't hurt anyone, overconsumption of alcohol dilates the blood vessels of the face, leading to broken blood vessels. The result can be—in the extreme—a spidery red W. C. Fields type of nose, which is not exactly a hallmark of youthful innocence.

If you have this dilation problem (which can also be caused by spicy foods or exposure to extreme heat or cold), a dermatologist may be able to do away with these broken vessels by "sparking" them with high-frequency electric current, but there is a slight risk of scarring. Cryosurgery is a newer technique—the broken vessels are sprayed with liquid nitrogen, so there is no scar, but neither are results guaranteed. Still, many patients who have been drinking over the years are pleased with the results. But it's much better to avoid too much alcohol (especially as you pass the age of resiliency) and avoid the problem.

Alcohol also leads to wrinkles in two ways. First, it dehydrates your skin —and water loss leads to wrinkle gain. Second, it doesn't allow your system to metabolize the vitamins you take via pills or food, so your skin becomes poorly nourished. You don't see cosmetics manufacturers looking for models on Skid Row!

You'll age too soon without smoking or alcohol—why give yourself more wrinkles than are necessary?

Can anything be done about the vertical scowl lines between my eyebrows . . . they make me look angry, even when I'm not.

I spoke of two major categories of removable wrinkles, the life-style overload—too much smoking, drinking (and too many late nights), and environment-induced lines. You've just asked me about another—"expression wrinkles." These are lining patterns we do unto ourselves; they have nothing to do with age. Remember, *if it's not age-related, it doesn't have to be there.*

IF YOU	THEN YOU HAVE
wrinkle your forehead, raise your eyebrows	horizontal forehead grooves
knit your brows when thinking, angry	scowl line
squint	crow's-feet
smoke	premature wrinkles above upper lip, around eyes
tug on eyes when applying eye make-up	drooping eyelids
chew on upper/lower lip	curved lines surrounding mouth

Does this mean you should strive for an immovable masklike effect? Not unless you're on exhibit like King Tut—and he's been *dead* for some 3,000 years. You just have to cut out the *quirky* little movements that probably detract from your appearance.

If you stop your harmful expression habits, this will prevent further damage, even though it won't soften the lines that are already there. For that, you need intensive treatment, which you'll learn about in Part Three, the Stay-Young Workshop.

℞. *Foolproof Facial Mannerisms Test.* Take a piece of hair-setting tape and place it over the wrinkled areas on your face. See how often the tape tightens as you go about your daily routine when you are home (doing this in public will definitely get you a seat on the bus—and one for your shopping bag, too). If the tape tightens often, concentrate on not making the faces in question. It will take time and effort, but once you're aware of what your face is doing, you'll be able to control it.

SNEAK PREVIEW. Substitute Snip-and-Tuck Wrinkle Trainer (Chapter 5) for tape.

℞. *Nightwork.* If you're particularly tense and dream of being chased by men and horses (or *not* being chased by the former!), you could be scrunching up your face when you sleep . . . in which case, overnight taping of troubled areas may be in order.

℞. *To fight nighttime tension,* indulge in daytime exercise: Regular physical workouts help you sleep better. You should also sleep with a window open—fresh air is a natural soporific.

⸙ *Will all diets cause the skin to line and sag?*

Dieting itself isn't the culprit—it's how, and how often, you diet that can turn good intentions into bad habits.

Under the How

If your weight-loss program includes diet pills in the form of diuretics, you may experience too rapid a loss of water. While this will show on the scales as an ego-boosting weight loss, it will show on your face as dehydration—water loss from the cells will make you look prematurely lined and wrinkled. Since diuretic-induced weight loss is only temporary but its effects on your skin may be long-lasting, avoid it.

How Often

If you lose 10 pounds one month, gain it back plus a few extra the next month, drop 15 six months later, you're courting skin disaster. When you gain weight, the added fat causes your skin to stretch to cover the enlarged area. When you lose weight suddenly, that excess facial (and body) skin has nothing to hang on to . . . so it creases into wrinkles, sags into bags.

This *doesn't* mean you should carry around 10 pounds of excess flab for the sake of your skin! It does mean you have to take off weight in a healthful manner (starving it off leaves your skin starving for nourishment, too) and provide your skin with the vitamins and water it needs to undergo the "shock" of losing all that *avoirdupois*. And you must resolve to keep it off. *It's the yo-yo diet plan that wreaks havoc with your complexion.*

Can dieting be *good* for the skin? In Chapter 7, I'll explain how to lose 2 to 5 pounds in 24 hours *healthfully* (really! you can!), plus I'll explain how to add just one ingredient to your favorite diet that will help you avoid that lean-and-mean look forever.

REMEMBRANCE OF SKIN PROBLEMS PAST

My 30th birthday has brought with it a few dry skin lines and some crow's-feet, but I still get occasional blackheads and some pimples. What to do?

Post-puberty breakout is not uncommon, especially if you had oily skin to begin with. When your no longer alabaster-smooth complexion breaks out, all skin imperfections, including minor lines, seem to stand out—so you look older than you should. The problem: how to curb blemishes without promoting wrinkles. Most over-the-counter blemish-control agents on the market are made for *teen-age* skin. They contain strong drying ingredients like resorcinol, sulfur, or salicylic acid. If you still find these effective and you're old enough to remember the "Clearasil personality of the month" ad campaign (wherein a girl's acne miraculously cleared the afternoon of the sockhop), apply sparingly. Dilute with water if you peel too much, and modify usage directions, starting with half the daily recommended dose: You can always work your way up.

℞. *If your breakout problems are confined to the T-zone areas* (forehead, nose, and chin), a commercial peel-off might suit you to a "T." Many companies make these nonchemical peeling products containing waxes that combine with other ingredients and declog your pores by dislodging the oil plug whose surface turns into a blackhead when the oil hits the air.

℞. *Don't use an anti-acne soap*—it's too hard to control lather placement. And since oil-clogged pores, rather than dirt, cause pimples and blackheads, washing your face with harsh acne-fighting soap thrice daily won't eliminate breakouts. It *will* produce unnecessary dry skin wrinkling.

℞. *Treat only the affected area of your skin with blemish lotion.* Dot on the pimple with a Q-tip; don't swab all over your face.

✺ *As a teen-ager in the late 50s, I "slinked" around imitating Marilyn Monroe in every way. I even wore heavy pancake make-up, yet I never had a pimple. As a clean-living, healthy-eating woman of the 70s, I now have a breakout problem.*

It sounds as if you have what doctors call adult acne (I call it the Messy Skin Syndrome), which is more common than you think. Messy skin can occur *anytime* from puberty to menopause; the grown-up variety seems to afflict the lower half of the face and neck most severely. If you have a serious case, you want to take immediate action—there's no point in waiting to outgrow it. And when it comes to skin, I define "serious" as anything that makes you unhappy—although the regular occurrence of three blemishes during your period shouldn't cause you to transfer your savings to a skin specialist. Dermatologists use antibiotics (tetracycline, erythromycin, clindamycin), vitamin A acid applied directly to your skin, and assorted drying lotions.

℞. *Test any prescribed lotions on a small area first*, checking for parching side effects. You don't want a blemish lotion turning your skin into a ringer for crazed porcelain. (Surely the term "crazed porcelain" was invented by a female potter! When my skin took on this overly dry "antiqued" look in patches, I *felt* as crazed as I looked.)

℞. *It could be "contact" acne.* Your fingers shouldn't touch your face. Exception: You've washed your hands in preparation for your face exercises.

When you're alone, put a piece of hair-setting tape under your chin—it will serve as an anti-touch alarm button if you often cup your chin in your hand.

℞. *If you work with carbon paper, don't touch your face.* Carbon turns more than your fingertips black; it can also turn your face red—by causing it to break out.

Messy Skin Syndrome: The Stress Factor

While some doctors drone on about adult acne and blocked pores, most women in their 30s with moderate skin problems don't understand that the true *underlying* cause is really stress. Yes! Stress throws your hormones out of balance and turns normally docile sebaceous glands into "superglands" that spew oil faster than a newly struck gusher.

Look to your current life situation for the reasons why. Are you suffering through a sticky divorce; suffering under a career strain; suffering with the reality that you're tied to a less-than-storybook mate; or suffering from the "empty nest" syndrome (your kids no longer need you the way they used to)? Your skin reflects your inner health, and when you try to break out of a messy situation, your complexion "breaks out" too. All the resorcinol in the world won't help—you have to look to your inner resources and take even better care of yourself when tense. *Force* yourself to get enough food, sleep, exercise, and vitamins. It's the only way to compensate for hyperactive adrenal glands.

Stress also causes premature age lines—removable wrinkles—which we can all do without. If you lose sleep, don't eat properly, and walk around with a perpetual frown, you will find yourself looking older. The resulting state of your skin will probably further aggravate your fragile nerves. It's a fact that supremely happy people usually have clearer, more unlined skins than average. Luckily for the rest of us, there are few of these paragons of joy around for comparison purposes.

The Pill

Your messy skin could be caused by something as mundane as the birth control pill you're taking. Women ingesting a formula heavy in progesterone (the male hormone) may notice more frequent breakouts, which changing to a pro-estrogen pill just might cure. Ask your doctor.

SIGNS OF TIME

🌑 *I want to try to avoid face "future shock." What wrinkles can I expect to appear, and when? And, can I keep them from appearing?*

There is only one way of preventing all signs of facial aging indefinitely—die young! To live is to line, but that doesn't mean your face has to look as tracked as Churchill Downs after the Kentucky Derby. It is more than possible to delay the onset of many lines, eliminate some altogether, and camouflage the rest practically until your dotage. You can have terrific skin during your in-between years, your 30s . . . 40s . . . 50s, the best part of your life, by following specific skin regimens set forth in this book.

But what if you ignore the Beat-the-Clock Skin-Care System you will learn in Part Three and trust your future face to fate—not to mention to the same soap you've used since you first learned to buckle your own Mary Janes? I don't have to look too deeply into my crystal ball to predict the results of laissez-faire/no-care skin care.

The Future Shock Face Change Chart

Age 25–30: The beginning of laugh lines, a term more often used by women in their 20s, because young women really don't think of themselves as aging (the "what, me worry?" syndrome). Minor lines and wrinkles at this point are called expression lines or dimples—but the dimples are starting to spread, and they don't go away when you stop smiling.

Age 30–35: Those facial changes are no longer solely in your imagination. There's a slight sagging, the undereye may look a bit puffy, crow's-feet appear. Those who love you say you still look 16, because the telltale signs aren't that obvious, but your "expression lines" are now deepening. If you go to a dermatologist for help, he usually looks at you skeptically, and you feel as though you should have the word "vain" etched into your forehead in salicylic acid.

(If you choose to tell a little white lie about your age, you can get away with it from 25 to 35, if you're so inclined. It's very difficult for someone to guess whether you're 27 or 32. From 32 to 35, it remains difficult . . . *if* you take care of your skin.)

Age 35–40: Those loving friends who claimed you didn't look a day over 16 when you were 34 suddenly ask, "My God, what *happened* to you?"

Like a blouse that's been worn once, you're not completely wrinkled, but you no longer have that fresh, smooth look. Your expression lines may now become frown lines if you're not careful.

Age 40–45: Your skin isn't just creasing, it's folding and sagging, and you may notice tiny cross-hatched wrinkles above your upper lip and under your eyes. If you've spent the last 20 years cultivating a drop-dead tan, your face will look as if it's already interred.

Age 45–50: Face falling and sagging continues, deepening of expression lines occurs. But your face can still look firm and moist if you know how to handle it and don't neglect nourishing treatment creams. You may notice a drop in the lower half of the face, a double chin, and the tendency to jowls. The shape of your neck will make you haunt the turtleneck sweater rack, and you may start noticing wrinkles on the backs of your hands.

Age 50+: More wrinkles and sagging; skin that's been subjected to a lifetime of neglect takes on a yellowed, parched, malnourished look.

The foregoing predicts what *could* take place on your face . . . but it's *not* inevitable. Careful attention to this and the next chapter and the Stay-Young Workshop can delay the possibilities in each category *for up to 10 years!*

The rest of this chapter will answer questions about specific *Signs of Time* that may be making their first appearance on your face.

Down in (and around) the Mouth (and Chin, Throat)

I've noticed a few vertical lines above my upper lip. They look like tiny cuts. I'm still young, but I'm worried.

One thing you *can't* do: have a face-lift. It just won't correct this problem, which, like many others, unfortunately afflicts women more than men. According to Dr. Auerbach, whom we mentioned earlier, these fine, cross-hatched wrinkles extending upward and outward from your upper lip occur because of heredity and sun damage. The best way to fill in these lines: Have a qualified doctor inject minute amounts of silicone into the wrinkles.

Your mouth area wrinkles may be caused by a source you never suspected—your teeth! Tooth problems (including lack of a tooth or two) can make a woman in her 30s or 40s look much older (not to mention much less attractive). Advances in cosmetic dentistry can change many of these problems (and wrinkles) from permanent to removable. Because it's such an important subject, I discuss cosmetic dentistry more fully in the next chapter.

Another reason your above-lip looks wrinkled: You may be suffering from a syndrome known as "the shrinking upper lip," which stalks every woman after she passes the nymphet stage. To compensate:

℞. *Perform do-it-yourself skin peels* on the lip area twice weekly if you have above-the-lip lining. Commercial at-home peeling products give a mild peel and, of course, there are no penetrating chemicals to worry about.

℞. *Perform a make-it-yourself "salabrasion."* Mix 1 tablespoon sea salt with 1 cup of hot (not boiling) mineral water. Wait until it cools a bit, then rub it gently over the affected area for a sea-based, safe skin peel.

Whoever named those mouth-to-nose rivers "laugh lines" must have a warped sense of humor. Mine look like deep furrows, yet the rest of my face is fairly smooth. What can I do about them?

First, don't stop laughing and smiling. There are good expression lines that indicate you're not an android, and smiling is one of them. To keep the good from becoming annoyingly obvious, get out your eye oil or under-eye stick and dab over expression lines a few times a day. This will soften their appearance, and the exercises I will teach you will firm the naso-labial support structures, which is what laugh lines really are. Make-up can help, too—see Part Six.

God said everyone gets one of everything—yet I've been "blessed" with two chins.

Two chins *are* too much of a good thing . . . and much too common. You don't have to be old or fat to possess a double chin; you can be young and thin—with poor posture. If you walk with your head slumped forward and your chin practically resting on your neck, your chin will look as doubled over as your shoulders (you're also a double-chin candidate if you spend the day hunched over your desk or typewriter).

There's another chin-area problem: the turkey wattle or dry, crepey neck with a hanging, flapping-in-the-wind fold of flesh. This can be improved in other ways than merely by wearing a turtleneck. The neck/throat area contains no oil glands, yet your regular *lubricating* cream alone won't help. You need a cream specifically labeled for the throat that contains tightening agents as well as emollients. Apply with sweeping upward and outward massage movements. You must also couple your double-chin workout with the exercises you will learn to strengthen the neck muscles your downtrodden posture has made lax.

And there's one more caveat. Sudden, unhealthful dieting, while it may take off the weight, will also leave your skin overly stretched, without permitting it to rejuvenate itself. The result: too much flesh with nothing to anchor itself to, a special problem in the neck region of yo-yo dieters.

℞. *To whittle a double chin,* keep your lower jaw muscles working. Chewing something tougher than spaghetti will help your chin line as well as your middle. Munch on carrot sticks, celery, apples (the latter two are also natural breath fresheners). Use exaggerated mouth movements—feel your jaws work with each bite.

℞. *Make your own throat cream* by simply adding ¼ teaspoon alum to an 8-ounce jar of cold cream. Alum is a tightening agent (find it in the drugstore). Massage tightening cream into your breasts, too. The bosom treatment is an important salon service in Europe; I'll give you a super at-home version in the Stay-Young Workshop to come. After all, you don't want firm, young-looking skin to end at your neck!

Beware the "Eyes" of March

Since neither Shakespeare nor anyone else has written sonnets praising crow's-feet and such, the following Q's and A's may interest you.

I have the normal amount of crow's-feet for a 30-year-old; what can I do to keep them from getting worse?

You're a candidate for a good eye oil, which you should apply liberally 3 or 4 times a day. The point is to keep the undereye and crow's-feet skin moist all the time. You want a lightweight eye oil, one that can be applied both under and over make-up without ruining it or making you look greasy. An eye *cream* is usually thick and "tacky" and won't penetrate as well as an oil combo. I actually keep my eye oil in my desk or in my pocket, so I can reapply it a few times daily, whenever I think of it. Pat the oil into place, don't rub or tug.

There are no oil glands on your eyelids, and lid skin is a mere one millimeter thick (just about the thinnest on your body) . . . two good reasons to keep the area, as well as the crow's-feet, thoroughly moisturized. (You might find a line-softening stick more convenient. These contain lubricants like castor oil and lanolin housed in a lipstick-type tube; you can apply the stick directly over make-up.)

℞. *At bedtime,* pat eye oil on your upper lid, too.

℞. *Quit smoking.* As I mentioned earlier, there is a definite causal relationship between crow's-feet and smoking. If you don't want your "feet" to spread into a sunburst pattern, break this bad habit.

⬙ *I wake up in the morning and my eyelids look so puffy. Why, and what can I do about it?*

Puffy lids give rise to the "Incredible Shrinking Eye" (an ever-smaller opening surrounded by ever-more-hanging flesh), and since a wide-eyed look is a sign of youth, you want to minimize puffs. First, you have to determine the cause; it may be more a health problem than a cosmetic defect. Certain allergies, as well as sinus problems, cause fluids to pool in the eyelids; a doctor can prescribe medication to counteract the condition and the resultant fluid build-up. But before you see an allergist, do a little sleuthing yourself. Make sure whatever products you're using to lubricate the eye area at night (I hope you're using something) aren't leading to an allergic reaction.

If puffs disappear as the day wears on, the pooling could be caused by water retention, which occurs as we lie prone at night and tends to get worse as we get older. Why do water-filled puffs disappear in the daytime? As we go about our daily activities in an (hopefully) upright posture, the water simply drains out of our eyelids.

℞. *If you can't wait* half a day for your puffs to drain, sleep with a couple of extra pillows tucked under your head to give you all-night elevation.

℞. *Keep a stock* of camomile tea bags soaked in ice water in the fridge; apply tea bags to your puffs for 10 minutes when the alarm rings. Not only will you be invigorated, but the astringent bags should help temporarily reduce the swelling.

℞. *To minimize the possibility of an adverse reaction to eye oil*, make sure you don't pat the oil on too close to the eye—blurred vision is not your goal! If oils bother you, switch to the stick form; the wax base will keep the oils from sliding into your eyes.

℞. *Study the "puffy eye" make-up cues*, Part Six.

Here are some other eye-area problems that need discussion:

Crepey, Wrinkled Skin on Upper and Lower Lids

Because the skin in this area is so thin, it doesn't contain much melanin to protect the collagen fibers from sun damage. Nor does it contain much collagen to begin with, and the amount found in the eyelids is moved so often (much more than cheek skin, say) it collapses earlier than the rest of the face. Combine this collapsing-collagen problem with the fact that there are no oil glands in this region, and you've got the makings of early wrinkles. To keep your lid area from aging you, make sure you keep it moist via nightly applications of your carefully chosen eye oil, which you should apply to both lids as well as the crow's-feet section beneath the lower lids.

Since today's squint lines are tomorrow's premature wrinkles, don't let misplaced vanity about glasses cause wrinkles. I will discuss glasses later.

Undereye Bags

These are different from puffiness, because they don't go away when you walk around or take medication. Often hereditary in nature, they can make their decidedly unwelcome appearance when you're still quite young —in your 20s. Yo-yo-type weight gain and loss is a factor; so is life style. If you can't fit sleep into your schedule but do find the time for alcohol, don't be surprised at seeing excess baggage under your eyes. These pouches are actually pockets of fat—herniated fat pads—that push through the eyelids' delicate and thin support structure till they form noticeable bulges. If a more Spartan life style doesn't reduce them, you may want to consider blepharoplasty—eyelid plastic surgery. In this procedure, the surgeon lifts the skin and muscle covering the "bag" and removes a portion of the fat pad found beneath. The doctor must be skilled in this procedure—eyelid skin is just one millimeter thick, and mistakes could impair the protective function of the lids. The stitches will be removed in about 5 days; the swelling usually subsides in 10 days, and if the job is well done, the stitches shouldn't be noticeable. Excess skin can also be removed from your upper lid. A blepharoplasty can be performed as part of a face-lift or separately.

Droopy Eye

The sad-eyed-lady look comes about when your eyebrow and upper lid both seem to fall floorward. As we start putting some distance between our current status and our 30th birthday, the eyebrows that heretofore rested comfortably above the bony ridge that's their natural home begin to fall, sometimes below the ridge. You can correct this problem with make-up, by learning how to reshape your brows via some do-it-yourself brow-lift tricks. See Part Six, for details.

If the outer corner of your upper lid is falling, giving your eyes that hooded lizard effect, you can make up for the deficiency with some clever make-up adaptations, which I will tell you about later. I believe the make-up artist's brush can be as important a youth tool as the cosmetic surgeon's scalpel—and it's certainly cheaper—but hooded lids do respond well to surgery: See the blepharoplasty description above.

CHAPTER 3

❦❦❦

Your Personalized
Skin-Rescuing Counterattack

Now that you are familiar with the major skin battle zones, you want to learn how to care for your face and zero in on particular trouble areas. But before you begin your hand-to-face combat, you must be certain of your current skin type.

Precisely because you live with your skin day in and day out, you're not aware of the subtle changes taking place within (and upon) it, so you don't change how you cope with them. Many women with so-called normal skin feel they can go on forever using a moisturizer and a bit of blusher, but normal skin can imperceptibly turn to dry as you pass 30, and to keep it normal you have to turn on the nourishment. You know you have dry skin? Fine, but the methods of dealing with dehydration may have changed since you made this discovery.

Hopefully, I've got you running to your magnifying mirror, ready to look deep into your pores. What should you look for? The following admittedly subjective skin-type test may tell you what you need to know—even if you'd rather not know it.

THE GRIM TRUTH SKIN ANALYSIS

On a separate sheet of paper, answer True or False to the following, then compare your responses with the analysis that follows to learn what kind of skin you're really in.

1. My face is so lined I should star in one of the Hope-Crosby road movies . . . as the map. My skin bears an uncanny resemblance to a road map of Morocco. True or False

2. When I touch my skin, I feel as though I have cellulite of the face—it's still lumpy and bumpy though I no longer look like a poster girl for an anti-acne campaign. True or False

3. I've inherited my mother's hot Latin blood and my father's propensity to cook with olive oil—I've nary a wrinkle, but I still have a case of forehead and nose greasies (not to mention an identity crisis). True or False

4. After just one half hour in the sun, I look as though I should be served with a dish of drawn butter. True or False

5. After a full day in the sun, I imagine I'm being followed by a ukulele-strumming quartet humming "Lovely Hula Hands." It's not sunstroke—my skin turns a golden Hawaiian tan. True or False

6. My cheeks feel cracklin' dry when I smile; my nose, forehead, and chin are so oily you can see your reflection in them. True or False

7. I'm only 25, yet teen-agers take one look at my face and get up to give me a seat on the bus. True or False

8. My sweet 13-year-old daughter is dating the local marijuana dealer/garbage collector (pick one or combine for premature wrinkles); my husband has romantic dinners with his boss, a Sophia Loren/Cary Grant look-alike (pick one). If this isn't acne, they should name a disease after what I've got. True or False

Analysis

If you answered questions 1, 4, and 7 *True*, you truly have dry skin. If you answered 2, 3, and 5 *True*, you still have oily skin—but remember, this state of affairs (like most affairs) won't last forever, especially if you keep spending time in the sun. (Today's golden girl is tomorrow's old crone.) If you answered *True* to number 6, you have combination skin—and must treat it accordingly. If you answered *True* to number 8, you don't have to give up or join the Harper Valley PTA. You're suffering from the Messy Skin Syndrome, and you'll learn how to care for M.S.S. and the other skin types in the Beat-the-Clock Skin-Care System outlined in the Stay-Young Workshop.

Now that you know your skin type, you will want to know what you face now and in the future. The following guide is taken directly from my training manual—it's the behind-the-scenes skin-study information we give our facialists in my salons.

How Time Changes Basic Skin Types

OILY SKIN	POSSIBLE PROBLEMS
Coarse Texture and Large Pores	Feels rough to the touch.
"Greasy" Finish	From age 25 on, the persistent all-over-your-face shine will be confined to your nose, chin, and forehead. For every 5 years past age 25, subtract one oily zone. Your outer cheeks will dry first, your forehead second.
Messy Skin Syndrome	Expect the area that broke out when you were a teen-ager (and has lain dormant since) to erupt again if stress sets in.
Absorbs Make-up	The oil in the skin tends to "drink up" make-up. Sometimes it may cause make-up to change color. Because you're no longer completely oily, you'll notice uneven make-up changes: color in some areas, not in others. Your T-zone is especially prone to oil breakthrough/inadequate coverage.
Attracts Soil	Patches of your face attract dirt and grime. Skin stays cleaner a shorter time than other types.
Stays Young Longer	The natural oils in this skin type keep it free from lining and wrinkling longer than dry or combination skin.

COMBINATION SKIN	POSSIBLE PROBLEMS
[Often begins in mid-20s, when oily skin begins to get dry areas]	
Dry Cheek Area with Small Pores	Dry area may have some flakiness, especially as skin becomes less oily in transition to maturity. Post-25 combination skin may also add a wrinkle or begin to line under eyes and between nose and mouth.
Oiliness in Center of Face	The forehead, nose, and chin tend to have oiliness and enlarged pores. May be marked with blackheads and occasional blemishes as well as slight lines under eyes or on forehead, causing confusion as to correct skin type.

DRY SKIN	POSSIBLE PROBLEMS

[All your life you've probably been told you have beautiful, translucent skin. Since you've always taken bows for your complexion, it will be difficult to adjust to the changes that will begin to appear between 25 and 35. Dry skin needs the most care during this transition period.]

Refined Texture, Dull Finish	Pores are fine, skin is thinner than other types.
Flakiness	Dry, flaky skin most prevalent in mature dry skin, when pores recede.
Lines and Wrinkles	Dry skin loses its elasticity earlier—visible lines and wrinkles appear under eyes, across forehead, and between mouth and nose on young women.
Parched Appearance or Feel	Becomes especially taut after cleansing or exposure to sun and wind.
Occasional Breakout	In younger dry skin, blemishes occur because of menstruation, allergies, or nervousness, not oiliness.
Crepiness	Folds under the chin, occurring in mature dry skin.

WHAT TO USE AND HOW TO PERFORM THE SKIN-ESSENTIAL SIX

Your skin type is the clue that will help you decide which 10-years-off counterattack you should follow. A well-thought-out skin-care regimen includes certain basic steps. Every woman over the age of 18 should make the following part of her anti-wrinkle program: 1) Make-up removal; 2) Cleansing; 3) Sloughing; 4) Toning; 5) Balancing and Nourishing; 6) Stimulating and Firming. These six steps will counteract the effects time may have on your face.

But before I go through the steps, let me say a few words about product education, which is crucial if you are to maintain young-looking skin. If you use the wrong products, your skin certainly won't profit from the time you're spending to care for it. It doesn't much matter what's in the first lipstick you clandestinely smear on at age 12, but a knowledge of treatment products is critical if you're over 18. Yet very few women approach cosmetic counters knowledgeably, because consumer education is difficult to come by in the billion-dollar beauty business. Consider what follows your course in cosmetic treatment consumerism. After all, when you buy a sweater, you know the difference between acrylic and cashmere. It's even more important to understand what you're putting on your *face*.

Now I'll explain each step's importance to keeping your skin young and vital.

Step #1: Make-up Removal

Your skin type isn't the final determiner of your care regimen. What you put on your face (and how you take it off) counts, too. If you wear a full make-up (i.e., foundation, blusher, eye make-up), it will take special care to remove every trace of it.

Normal to oily skins should cleanse twice daily with a soap replacement liquid (more about these shortly) to remove make-up. Two gentle cleansings are better than one strong lots-of-elbow-grease lathering.

If your skin is normal to dry, use cold cream, which is really a specially designed make-up melt, a solvent formulated to clear your skin of cosmetic remnants before cleansing. Put it on, leave in place one minute (so it has a chance to dissolve your make-up), and remove with a wet washcloth. Don't push and pull the washcloth around your face: Just pat it around and it will soak off dissolved make-up as well as the melt.

Proper make-up removal will add just an extra minute to your care routine, but it can help keep the years from showing on your skin, especially if your complexion is on the dry side. Why? Because melts are designed to glide across your skin without any "drag"—so you needn't push around the gentle collagen fibers to remove stubborn make-up.

Step #2: Cleansing

You rejuvenate your skin by removing accumulated dirt, pollution, and dead surface skin cells. Soap, the most common choice (made from animal fat, water, and an alkaline substance—usually salt—for cleansing), should not be used. Soap itself isn't *aging* (only birthdays are aging), but its inherent alkalinity, which gives it the power to de-dirt your skin, makes it *drying*—so unless you have a super-oily complexion, I don't recommend soap. (If you are stuck on soap, rinse *extremely* well so no traces will stick to your face. Soap residue promotes that tight, dry feeling.)

You are truly oily? You can try to control (though never completely) soap's drying tendency by checking out the ingredients before you check out the product on your skin. Unless you're an acne sufferer too young to vote, avoid soaps containing resorcinol, salicylic acid, tar, or sulfur.

If you still have oily skin and occasional breakouts, but you've also noticed your first laugh line, don't use just any supermarket soap. Of course, you know you must avoid the acne-scourge formulas, but there are ingredients that will help you. Look for a soap containing mild cleansing grains, or consider a non-soap cleanser containing natural minerals, tiny particles of sea kelp and/or pumice (a gritty combo of alum and alkali metals of volcanic origin) to do your cleansing.

If you have slightly to very dry skin and are over 30, you're doing your future face a definite disservice if you're stuck on soap. There is a whole world of alternate cleansers out there, including foaming soap-replacement-liquid (S.R.L.) cleansers that are greaseless and rinse off with water . . . and emollient-rich cleansers in cream form that will extract dirt without leaving a residue. If you're very dry, try the latter category; slightly oily to slightly dry will do well with S.R.L. cleansers. Some ingredients these two types of non-soap cleansers may contain: laneth-5 (a lanolin derivative) and stearic acid/decyl oleate (coconut derivatives) for softening and smoothing skin; allantoin (a healing agent); papain enzyme (derived from the papaya—it's a keratolytic agent, i.e., it sloughs off dead skin); citric acid to balance the pH. Precisely because they are in foam or cream form, they contain emollients (like mineral oil, lanolin, etc.), so your skin feels smooth as well as clean—none of that post-wash flaky texture that soap leaves behind.

If you've been blessed with normal skin since you left the cradle, just remember that today's problem-free complexion will definitely become drier as you add more candles to your birthday cake, so be prepared to adapt your cleansing routine as you head down the road a piece.

While I'm saying a few paragraphs about cleansing, let me talk about water. No matter what form of skin cleanser you use, make sure your face is wet before applying, and don't rinse in hot water. Super-hot water opens your pores. An open pore is like an open faucet—it lets the water drip out. So, though you may not see it, the hotter the water, the greater the chance of dehydration. A closed pore is a sealed pore; it keeps water and oil in their place, on your skin, so rinse in tepid or cool (not icy cold) water. (Reminder: Cleansing specifics for your skin type will be found in the Beat-the-Clock Skin-Care System to come. So will how-tos for the steps that follow.)

Step #3: Sloughing

Your skin will tell you how often to include this step in your care routine. If your complexion is very dry and sloughing daily makes your face look and feel like a raw wound, you're overdoing. Remember, that top layer of skin keeps your insides from flying through the air . . . you don't want to slough right down to your dermis. If you have fine surface wrinkles and your skin looks dull and ashen, see how your complexion reacts to twice-weekly sloughing. Your cheeks are dry but your T-zone rivals that of your preteen daughter? Spot slough: 3 times a week in the T; once a week on the rest of your face. Every woman needs to slough; you determine how often by studying your skin type and the feel of your skin. Men don't need to slough—they remove cellular debris during their daily shave; some credit for the younger look and feel of older men's skin must go to the lowly razor.

No matter how and with what you exfoliate the skin, you have to follow up with a rehydration routine: Splash 10 times with warm water and pat dry, leaving skin slightly damp. Keep skin soft and supple by finishing your slough-and-rinse with the application of a water-retaining moisturizer.

You're worried that all this sloughing will make dry skin drier? Don't be. You're only manipulating the very top layer of your skin—the layer that's old, dead, and has been hanging around for too long anyway. You're certainly not reaching down to your skin's moisture-producing apparatus in the dermis. Don't overdo the procedure, and do remember to rehydrate and moisturize as soon as you've finished. If you're very dry and have such sensitive skin that it hurts to smile, let alone exfoliate, you may be better off performing the ritual once every two weeks.

FLASHBACK: See earlier part of chapter for sloughing materials.

Step #4: Toning

Perform this quick pick-me-up ritual after cleansing, before moisturizing, to stimulate your skin, tighten your pores, make fine wrinkles less noticeable. Most women store away their skin toner with their senior prom corsage, and it's too bad. Even if your skin has a few wrinkles, the right toner can make it look smoother while adding zing to a dull complexion. By a *toner* I mean an astringent or skin freshener. Astringents are more powerful (i.e., more drying), but both types operate on the same general principle. The toner slightly irritates the skin. This minor irritation (what you feel as that delicious tingling sensation) causes the skin surrounding your pores to swell, thus blocking the pore opening from view. Enlarged pores are more of a problem as we get older, because the skin loses elastic tissue, thus the pores lose some of their ability to reclose. In the same way, skin surrounding finely etched surface wrinkles puffs up, causing these wrinkles to appear slightly less noticeable. The effects of these products are temporary, but you can always tuck your trusty toner into your bag for quick refreshing.

If your skin is normal to dry, choose a freshener: It will wake up your face and temporarily tighten pores without drying your skin.

If you have oily skin and are under 35, you can use an astringent . . . on one condition: You must dilute it to half strength with mineral water or rose water.

Step #5: Balancing and Nourishing

Yes, *balancing* (or moisturizing) does provide *some* lubrication for your skin by returning to the surface some of the oils lost in the cleansing and toning processes, but its main function is to seal in the skin's own natural moisture—water. In other words, your moisturizer serves as a barrier, helping prevent your skin's natural lubricant, H_2O, from leaching out into the air. A few words about applying your moisturizer:

Wet your skin first with water; pat dry to remove the excess only. With your skin still damp, gently dot on the moisturizer and spread lightly across skin. If you don't apply moisturizer to wet skin, you've got no water to lock in, so you're missing the barrier benefit of moisturizing. After applying, give it a minute or two to settle before continuing with your regimen.

If your skin type registers oily, you still need a moisturizer. First, because once skin starts showing a few laugh lines it is no longer completely oil-saturated from temple to jawline. Second, a moisturizer locks water inside your skin. You need this function performed no matter what form your skin surface takes. What you need is a moisturizing blotting lotion (many companies make them), a nongreasy preparation that combines lightweight oils with healing agents such as allantoin, which soothes the skin while promoting the growth of healthy new tissue.

℞. *Remoisturize when:*

◻ You're sitting near an open fire. Don't sit too close—the heat may break capillaries, causing tiny red "spider" veins to appear on your face.

◻ You plan on opening and closing the oven several times to baste or otherwise check your culinary endeavors.

◻ You're using your blow dryer or curling iron on a "hot" setting.

℞. *Don't moisturize your face when you bathe or shower.* Instead, apply your nourishing day cream; the heat and mist will help the cream penetrate, turning bath time into treatment time.

Nourishing refers to the addition of emollient, anti-aging treatment creams that use special ingredients to perform additional youth-retaining skin tasks. Together, the right Balancing and Nourishing routine will keep your face from looking like the bark on a sturdy oak tree.

Let's take it from the top and get to the bottom of the moisturizer–treatment cream maze. Why should you bother with a moisturizer, day and night cream, eye oil, throat cream? Because they're really underwear for your face. Put another way: How does an over-30 woman look in a slinky, satiny Jean Harlow gown without hold-me-in, push-me-up undergarments? Not too terrific. A young girl can get away with wearing nothing underneath; we can't. The same thing goes for skin. First the undergarments—moisturizers and so forth—then the frosting, the make-up.

Why do you need a *set* of nourishing treatment products? A quick study of your own body will confirm that the skin in different areas has a different thickness, texture, and feel—so it must be handled differently. If you come across a bottle full of miracles (i.e., one cream that touts itself as the solution for *all* skin problems), keep looking. If you're not ready to purchase your treatment regimen in one fell swoop, buy in the following order: 1) eye oil, 2) day cream, 3) night cream (Note: In the next chapter you'll learn how to make Prescription Sleep Serums—super night treatments tailored to specific skin problems), 4) throat cream.

Step #6: Stimulating and Firming: Masks

No matter what your skin type or condition, you will receive a definite complexion boost if you become a regular devotee of masks. These oldest of beauty aids have been adding zing to lethargic skins since Cleopatra first went barge-hopping with Mark Antony.

You will use a mask to stimulate and firm your skin, temporarily tighten the pores, help heal blemishes, and/or plump up wrinkles. The two main mask categories are gel and clay (or mud—depending on which copywriter is creating the description). Broadly speaking, gels are for dry skin, clay/mud for oily. (There are also subcategories, such as a spearmint mask, which would work for normal to oily skin but is not as strong as mud.) You will have no trouble distinguishing each type by its look and feel.

Here's how masks work: The mask-induced tingle your skin feels means your blood circulation is being stimulated, which in turn gives your face a nice rosy glow when you "unmask." Your surface lines will be less noticeable because (like toners) masks produce a slight irritation that not only refines enlarged pores—it also plumps up the skin surrounding your wrinkles, so they may appear temporarily to disappear. Your complexion will look smoother, clearer, and fresher because the mask will dislodge the dead, flaky cellular debris that gives skin a gray pallor and reduces complexion clarity.

Clay/mineral/mud masks work to draw off surface oils as well and are deep-cleansers. *Messy skin*, even if dry, can benefit from clay's ability to lift out grime, blackheads, and whiteheads. Once clay helps clear your messy, dry skin, switch to a gel. If you have *oily skin*, you'll want to make a clay mask part of your beauty arsenal.

Gels don't have oil-drawing properties. They help lock in moisture, so they're for the normal to dry skinned.

Combination skin? Cosmetic saleswomen say you'll need both types of masks. But if you don't want to buy two, stick with the milder one and you'll still be serving your skin well.

Masks also provide a psychological lift: Because you have to keep your face immobile during treatment, you (hopefully) lie down . . . so you should feel as well as look rested and refreshed when the mask comes off.

℞. *Make sure you mask your throat* to tone and tighten this region.

℞. *Mask more often in hot weather* to remove dead skin build-up.

℞. *Smile before applying* so you see just how far your crow's-feet (if you have any) extend—avoid masking that area as well as the more immediate eye region, because the skin surrounding the eyes is too fragile to be subjected to the tightening action of even the gentlest of masks.

Sneak preview. Now that you know what to use and how to perform the skin-essential six, you may be asking yourself "how often?" Before I spell it all out for you in the Beat-the-Clock Skin-Care System in Part Three, I want to give you still more skin-saving advice in the next two chapters, which I will then show you how to incorporate into your Beat-the-Clock Skin-Care System.

But first, some advice from the medical professionals.

FROM THE MEDICAL BAG

If you find yourself losing some crucial skin battles even though you take proper care of your skin, you may have to call in the "heavy artillery," the beauty doctors, to make your 10-years-younger campaign a success. Here are Q's and A's relating to professional medical treatments.

I understand that surface wrinkles are generally caused by dehydration— water loss. How does a face-lift smooth away these wrinkles?

It doesn't, and that's why many women are disappointed by their surgery. A face-lift will help you remove baggy, jowly skin; it will raise and tighten the skin that suddenly appears too big for your features, skin that has fallen as a result of age and gravity; it will make you look well rested.

But if you're also bothered by those fine, cross-hatched wrinkles that give your skin a dried-up appearance, a good plastic surgeon will recommend you schedule a chemical peel or dermabrasion following your surgery (these office procedures are usually performed by a dermatologist, sometimes by a plastic surgeon). In a chemical peel, the top, wrinkle-laden layer of your skin is burned off by the application of caustic chemicals. In dermabrasion, a rapidly rotating stainless steel wire brush is the tool. Your skin will peel/ crust/ooze for 10 days following the procedures, after which fresh young skin is revealed, giving you a plumper, smoother look.

You needn't be considering a face-lift to benefit from a dermabrasion or chemical peel. Many no-lift women visit their dermatologists twice a year for a mild peel that actually gets rid of finely hatched surface wrinkles . . . even crow's-feet. If done well, the recipient looks terrifically rested, refreshed, and rejuvenated, as if she's just had a two-week vacation (following her week to 10 days of self-imposed solitary confinement during the crusting period).

While these doctor-done abrasions *sound* like the best of all possible skin treatments, there are five points to consider.

Point #1: Skill

The dermatologist's skill is of utmost importance. If he or she wields the chemical brush or abrading tool like a house painter rather than an artist, you're in trouble. Understand that dermatologists specialize, too. The genius who got rid of your husband's fungal infection or the research-oriented TV pundit who sounds off on rare skin diseases may not be for you—you need a *beauty-oriented* dermatologist, and you have to ask around to find one. Satisfied friends are always the best source, or you can contact doctors associated with large teaching hospitals—there's no guarantee they're perfect, but at least they're at the top of the profession. Note: Most doctors prefer to abrade rather than peel; they have more control of the wire brush than of the caustic chemicals a peel requires.

Point #2: Skin Type

If you have thick, leathery, olive-toned, large-pored skin, these procedures may not be helpful.

Point #3: Temporary Effects

Understand that the dramatic improvement you first see—the plumpness that makes your skin look so smooth—is really due to swelling; as the swelling subsides, your skin won't look quite so young and unlined.

Point #4: Discomfort

Think about your pain threshold. Skin abrading and peeling are uncomfortable, though venerable, techniques. Women have been torturing themselves for centuries in the name of youth. One of the earliest "peels" on record: Concubines in Turkish harems would run past torches held by eunuchs. The heat from the flames would definitely peel off the skin. Drastic, yes—but if the Pasha's passion waned, it was back to the fig fields!

Point #5: Pigment Changes

Some doctors say (though not often for publication) that if you have a peel/abrasion, the pigment never comes out perfectly even all over your face, and you may have trouble handling the sun. Still, most women do see an improvement, and if you're prepared to stay out of the sun as much as possible (you don't want a smooth, *mottled* complexion), this technique may serve your needs.

℞. *Questions to ask the doctor:*

- How will my skin type affect the results?
- How long will the results last?
- What will happen to . . . (point to the specific facial areas that bother you; ask what improvement you can expect so you won't be disappointed)?
- Which post-peel sunblock will be best for me . . . exactly how much sun can I take . . . and when?

Can silicone injections be used for wrinkles?

Though still controversial, in the right medical hands, injected in the right facial crevices, they can successfully fill in certain annoying wrinkles. The liquid silicone used must be pure medical grade, and so must the practitioner! And the wrinkles must be injected s-l-o-w-l-y and carefully. According to Dr. Robert Auerbach of New York University Medical Center, New York City, you can't expect results with just one office visit. Horizontal forehead lines may take anywhere from 12 to 24 treatments; vertical scowl lines between the eyebrows take less time than that; the nose-to-cheek smile lines may take 4 to 12 or 24 treatments, depending on whether these lines are fairly superficial or deep grooves. Even though a minuscule amount of silicone is injected in each session (1/300 oz. per visit, 1/10 cc for a face full of wrinkles each treatment), you should wait at least 3 to 4 weeks between office treatments, so you must be patient about results.

Drawbacks? If injected properly, there should be no pooling or problems with this inert material. Don't confuse face injections with breast injections; the latter are absolutely *verboten*—and for breasts, silicone (encased in plastic) is used in gel form rather than the liquid form used for the face.

I have a scar on my chin caused by an automobile accident a few years ago. The scar didn't bother me when it first happened, but now that my face is no longer puppy-young, this "red badge of courage" seems to stand out more than ever. Can I get rid of it?

One of the minor miracle arts of plastic surgery is scar revision, wherein the doctor can often take a broad, deeply pigmented scar and trade it in for a less noticeable hairline-thin version, or reposition the scar so it's hidden completely. Dr. Paul Striker, a Manhattan plastic surgeon, explains that scars on the forehead can often be hidden in the hairline; jaw-area scars can be tucked behind the ear.

In your case, a doctor might be able to lower your chin scar a bit so it would no longer show. If your scar was by the side of your mouth, the surgeon would try to reposition it in your naso-labial fold, or he may turn it into a horizontal line by your lip (where it would be less obvious, especially if you smile a lot).

A new incision is made, the damaged skin is lifted away from underlying tissue, and the old scar is cut off. The remaining skin is sewn back together so that it looks neater than the scar originally formed by Nature and is in a less conspicuous area. (If you were having a face-lift, scar revision could be done as part of it, but you don't need to schedule a lift to have a bothersome scar revised.)

Sometimes doctors are called upon to disguise the *cause* of a scar. It is not uncommon for a plastic surgeon to disguise the telltale wrist scars of an attempted suicide, for example, by changing the position and shape of the scars so they look as though they resulted from an indeterminate cause.

But scar revision is not a simple business. The location, size, and shape of the original scar, your skin type (thick, oily skins don't heal as well as thin, dry skins), and the surgeon's skill are all factors that will affect the outcome of attempts to make an unattractive scar less conspicuous.

You can also do some scar disguising yourself—with make-up. Cosmetic revision will often give you quite satisfactory results (see Part Six for details).

COSMETIC DENTISTRY

While the dentist's chair is about as popular a place to visit as the electric chair, proper attention to teeth and gums will put you in the catbird seat when it comes to fighting signs of aging. A practitioner skilled in *cosmetic* dentistry can use the latest techniques and materials to make you look younger and better (as opposed to just making sure your teeth don't separate from your gums!).

One thing is for sure: Bad teeth, lack of a tooth or two, or just an unappealing smile can age you. Keeping our special "in-between" years needs in mind, I asked Dr. Jack Stuart Kern, one of the foremost specialists in restorative and cosmetic dentistry (people in the entertainment field as well as businessmen and women from all parts of the world fly to New York just for his esthetic expertise), what in-between women can do to and for teeth and mouth to help us take 10 years from our faces. His report follows.

Dr. Kern's Cosmetic Dentistry Suggestions for the New In-Between Woman

℞ #1. *If you're unhappy with your teeth but are too embarrassed to wear braces* (you think they'd clash with your crow's-feet!), ask your dentist about alternatives.

For example, if you have slightly buck teeth and aren't ready for a "wired" smile, a dentist can actually cut off your protruding teeth at the gumline and replace them with caps that will be in perfect alignment. (Needless to say, capping takes less time than bracing.) Or he/she can adjust your bite. If your uppers are buck because your lower teeth push them out, it is sometimes possible for your lower teeth to be shortened so they no longer create pressure on your upper teeth the wrong way. Then you would only have to wear a removable retainer on your upper teeth (at night, when you sleep) until you achieve a more pleasing mouth profile.

What about irregular lower teeth that are all scrunched up together? The dentist can file the sides of the teeth so they will have room to be straightened, and the nighttime retainer will do the straightening.

If your only cosmetic defect is a small gap between your front teeth, it can be filled with an acrylic resin in just one dental trip, avoiding the need for caps or braces.

℞ #2. *Do opt for orthodontia* if your teeth really need adjustments that require braces. The ranks of adults who are walking around with braces are steadily growing (though the wire band is still metallic in color, the rest of the gear can now be made out of a not-so-visible plastic, which should be at least some small comfort).

After all, isn't six months or a year with braces a small price to pay for 20-plus years of straight teeth? If you have large gaps between your teeth, for example, you'll look younger (and amazingly better) when the spaces are closed up. Or if your teeth are lying willy-nilly overlapping each other (as unattractive as too widely spaced teeth), straightening will not only improve your smile, it will help you hold on to your teeth longer because there will be less compression on the gums. And healthier gums mean less tooth loss from gum disease.

℞ #3. *If you're in your 40s,* your teeth have been considerably shortened from the wear and tear of daily living, chewing (or grinding). As a result, your cheeks may appear a bit more sunken than is necessary and lines may form in the corners of your mouth. The dentist can restore your teeth to their original length with caps. This bite adjustment will increase the muscle tone in your cheek area, making your face look a bit fuller (and full equals young —except in the hip department!).

℞ #4. *If you're in your 50s* and have serious teeth problems that require the wearing of a denture, you can make the device do double duty by having it crafted in such a way that *it will actually fill out the wrinkles above your upper lip.* The flange (the plate that rests above the teeth—the pink-colored part that looks like gums) can be built out to support the lip, thus filling out the lines. It's also important for the denture teeth to be made the correct height (dentists talk about "vertical dimension"). If the teeth are too short, they won't support your face muscles, and you'll look older.

Note: You can't build out caps to support the upper lip. Caps that are too big and thick will only make you look ridiculous.

℞ #5. *Consider caps.* Crowns or porcelain jackets (other terms for caps) can give you the terrific smile you never had. For the best esthetic results, save up until you can do all six upper front-and-center teeth at once if needed. These are the teeth that really show—and they should all be the same color (it will be more difficult for the dentist to match them exactly if you do a couple now, a couple later).

Caps are not inexpensive, but they can go a long way toward making you look younger. For the top and bottom center six teeth, you usually can have solid porcelain jackets, but porcelain alone isn't strong enough for the back teeth, the biting surfaces. In the rear, you should have porcelain over a metal base (gold is best). In the back, gold crowns with a veneer of porcelain and an exposed gold biting surface would be best because they're strongest, but most women don't want any gold showing, so the most popular rear cap alternative is porcelain over gold (other nonprecious metals are used, but they're not as good as gold). All-plastic caps do exist, but they're not advisable front or back—acrylic changes color faster than porcelain and it's just not as strong.

℞ #6. *Replace lost teeth.* Periodontal disease, extensive decay, and tooth loss are all valid reasons for caps (or if necessary, dentures). If you don't replace lost teeth, your remaining teeth will wind up shifting around and loosening. Your whole bite may alter (to the detriment of your mouth, face, and remaining teeth).

Of course, if you don't take care of your teeth, you will have nothing left to beautify. Consider:

Dr. Kern's Dental Care Suggestions for the In-Between Woman

℞. #1. *If you're in your 30s*, start to worry about (and take care of) your gums. Brush and massage your gums with your soft-bristled toothbrush (dentists no longer recommend hard bristles) to stimulate circulation and toughen gums. Gum disease is responsible for more tooth loss after 40 than any other cause, including tooth decay. Some gum shrinkage is normal with age, but if your gums seem to be shrinking fast, see your dentist quickly. Shrinking gums lead to wobbly teeth, which lead to loss of teeth and spacing between teeth.

You should also use Stimudents (available in drugstores), little wooden sticks that you work around and between your teeth and gums after meals when you can't brush. These inexpensive "sons of the toothpick" will help you keep teeth/gums healthy by cleaning them and stimulating gum circulation. Flossing with unwaxed dental floss is also good for cleaning between teeth.

If your parents had gum disease, understand the problem may be hereditary, and you should take extra precautions. Regular curettage (gum treatments) performed by a competent dental hygienist and a diet rich in vitamin C and citrus fruits are important.

℞ #2. *If you're in your 40s*, your teeth may be starting to get brittle and yellowed with age. Yellowing occurs because the enamel wears out and the inside of your teeth (made of dentin, a yellowish substance) starts to show through. Don't use abrasive tooth powders or a hard toothbrush. Use soft bristles and brush your teeth (and gums) sideways, not up and down.

Periodic cleaning and avoiding cigarettes will help keep your teeth bright. Acrylic resins painted on the teeth can also brighten them. But whiter-than-white dazzlers may no longer be for you. Just as you have to adjust your hair color to your changing skin tone (you go for less bright, more subtle shades as you get older), so must you adapt your tooth color. If your dentist is an artist as well as an artisan, he may suggest a little more shading for most flattering results. You don't want *unnatural*, whitewashed picket-fence teeth.

℞ #3. *Brush your teeth and gums while in the shower*. Really! Most people are in a hurry when they brush their teeth, so they don't do a thorough job. But when you're in the shower, you're not going anyplace while the water is pounding down, so you can do the job properly.

℞ #4. *Don't think sugarless gum is okay*. It's awful, because gum (with or without sugar) gets stuck and breaks down between your teeth where it stays and decays. Dr. Kern says he'd rather see his patients eat sugar-rich chocolate than chew sugarless gum (though chocolate is not a recommended diet aid!).

℞ #5. *Don't grind your teeth*. If you are a nighttime gnasher (the condition is called bruxism) and you just can't quit, wear a night guard to bed (ask your dentist about fitting you with one). Otherwise your teeth will loosen, and you may eventually lose them.

❦❦❦

PART THREE

WELCOME TO MY STAY-YOUNG WORKSHOP

CHAPTER 4

❦❦❦

Prescription Sleep Serums:
The Precious Brown Bottle Collection

Now that you've donated your sun lamp to the local alchemist bent on transforming supple skin into old leather, and now that you understand you can no longer rely on tender teen-age collagen to keep your face young-looking, you're ready to take your complexion into your own hands.

Even Abraham Lincoln, an unlikely source of beauty advice, said that after the age of 40 a person is responsible for his own face.

But *you* become responsible for your own face, and the way it will (or won't) line, beauty-wise, when you blow out your 25th candle. To help you exercise your beauty responsibility with nothing less than Lincolnian wisdom (and to make sure you leave character and other forms of unnecessary lining to the "characters"), I've put together a collection of the savviest do-it-yourself anti-wrinkle treatments this (or that) side of a Swiss youth clinic, a veritable at-home skin science laboratory packed with effective complexion-saving regimens tailored for your face. This chapter is your first stop on my guided 10-years-off tour. We'll step into those super-sterile European labs where ingredients like vitamins, special oils, and secret additives are blended into precious formulas for the pampered few, formulas you will learn how to prepare for your own about to be richly pampered skin.

PRESCRIPTION SLEEP SERUMS:
THE PRECIOUS BROWN BOTTLE COLLECTION
DEFINED

Tucked away in tiny hamlets deep in the Swiss Alps are legendary chalets where you can take a "sleep cure." White-jacketed men and women keep the wealthy-but-corpulent-and-crinkled asnooze until they've lost weight/ purified their skins by not ingesting anything, toxic or otherwise. While I feel this is a radical (not to mention extremely boring) approach to beauty best left to those with loads of money whose presence won't be missed by anyone anyway (except perhaps by the local bank), you *can* work minor miracles on your skin while you sleep, *chez vous*. All you need do is create one or more of the following overnight sleep serums I developed with Dr. Albert Shansky, a famous consulting chemist, who was able to decode expensive European youth prescription creams and translate them into vitamin-packed formulas you can make in your own "lab" at home.

How to Create Your Own At-Home Skin Laboratory

INGREDIENTS

In a clean, well-lighted work space, assemble the following: a tray to hold your gear; a set of measuring spoons; 8- and 4-ounce amber bottles, which you can purchase from your drugstore (you want the amber-colored variety so the ingredients, including vitamins, will keep better; light attacks potency and freshness). You will also need a blender (to approximate the industrial homogenizers we use in our professional labs when we prepare treatment products similar to these for use in my salons). If your appliance won't pulverize tablets, add to your shopping list a mortar and pestle for easy crushing.

The rest of the ingredients you need for the serums—the vitamins and oils—can be obtained at your health food store or drugstore. Buy them in small quantities so they will stay fresh longer.

PREPARATION

The formulas following these how-tos are geared to a batch of both dry skin and oily skin complaints. Isolate the problem(s) that best describe the state of your face, and make the simple formulas according to the directions.

Before beginning your lab work, pour alcohol onto cotton and rub over your hands to sterilize them.

To make serums, prick open vitamin capsules and squeeze contents into blender; if your appliance won't pulverize tablets, use a mortar and pestle or grind between two spoons. Place ingredients in blender, whip till smooth consistency is achieved—about 15 seconds at low speed. Label and refrigerate dry skin, oil-based formulas overnight. Oily skin, mineral water–based formulas can be stored out of the fridge overnight.

Since these serums contain no preservatives, formulas will work better —and stay fresh longer—if made every other night. If you do want to make more than a two-night supply, you'll need a larger bottle, of course. But to help insure freshness, don't make more than enough for four nights at once.

APPLICATION

Consider the contents of your precious brown bottle a custom P.M. treatment, and use instead of a night cream. With your hair pulled back, apply to face (and throat if your neck region is starting to look less than smooth) with fingertips. Apply after application of your eye oil—just as you would your usual sleep cream. Apply 10 minutes before bedtime to give the serum a chance to sink into your skin (you want to treat your face, not your pillow!).

If you have more than one problem (who doesn't!), simply alternate treatment regimens: Stay with a formula designed to attack Problem #1 for two nights, switch to a second designed to attack Problem #2 for the next two nights, then return to the first.

Now you're ready to get to work. Serum prescriptions for dry skin problems are outlined first. Those for the oily side follow.

DRY SKIN SLEEP SERUMS: THE "MAGNIFICENT EIGHT" BASE

All of the dry skin serums share the following eight essential ingredients, which you will combine according to the formula that follows this descriptive listing:

□ *Mineral oil*—excellent lubricant derived from same base as petroleum jelly. Somewhat sticky to the touch, which means it's sticking to your skin.

□ *Castor oil*—hard-working, softness-producing emollient. Gives skin a moist look and feel. Castor oil makes up a third of most lipsticks. If it helps give lips (which become dry and cracked most easily if not protected) a smooth consistency, think what this terrific lubricator will do for your face.

□ *Lecithin*—a natural emulsifier that will keep your serum well blended. It is also rich in B vitamins and vitamin E.

□ *Cod liver oil*—one of the best sources of the skin vitamins, A and D. Keep it in the refrigerator so the vitamins won't lose their potency. Close bottle tightly to prevent oxidation.

□ *Gelatin*—derived from animal protein; an easily available collagen source.

□ *Seaweed or kelp*—mineral-loaded natural food, especially rich in iron (important for blood circulation, promotes good skin color) and magnesium (promotes cross-linkage of collagen, which leads to firmer skin—some cross-linkage is necessary, or your skin will look like clay that's been left out in the rain too long!). Kelp is also high in collagen-producing vitamin C.

□ *Multiple vitamin*—for multiple skin nutrition.

□ *Vitamin E*—a most important vitamin when applied externally to dry skin. Because it is very oily, it acts as a super line and wrinkle minimizer (dry-skinned devotees swear that lines look smoother after daily E applications). It also improves the circulation, helps heal scars. Body-plus for "yo-yo" dieters: E softens the appearance of stretch marks.

Formula for "Magnificent Eight" Base

1.	Mineral Oil	½ cup
2.	Castor Oil	1 tablespoon
3.	Lecithin	2 tablespoons
4.	Cod Liver Oil	½ tablespoon
5.	Unflavored Gelatin Preparation	½ cup
6.	Seaweed or Kelp	1 teaspoon
7.	Multiple Vitamin Tablet	1 tablet
8.	Vitamin E Capsule, 100 IU	1 capsule

To make, put first four ingredients in blender. To prepare gelatin: Dissolve 1 tablespoon gelatin in ¼ cup cold water; add ¾ cup boiling water to it. Allow to cool to body temperature and add ½ cup of the mix to blender (reserve remainder for use when preparing another serum). Add remaining ingredients.

The above "base" is an ℞ in itself *if you have rough, flaking, chapped-looking, always slightly red, thin skin.* If you have a more exotic dry skin problem, consult the ℞s and additives which follow.

℞. *If you have very wrinkled skin*, add 1 teaspoon sesame oil to base before blending.

Sesame is a rich source of natural vitamin E. Sesame oil has been used externally as a beauty oil for centuries. It also offers sun protection by blocking out about a third of the burning ultraviolets, so you may want to consider this serum for day use as well. Keep sesame oil refrigerated to prevent rancidity. The extra E in sesame oil, combined with the vitamin E in the formula base, will doubly smooth and soothe wrinkled skin.

℞. *If you have sun-damaged skin* (*brown spots, freckles*), add the gel of one Aloe vera leaf (or ¼ teaspoon dried Aloe vera powder) and one 1,000-mg PABA tablet to base before blending.

The water-rich Aloe vera plant has been used since biblical times to fight sunburn and sun damage. Aloe leaves are still used for these purposes in the Caribbean, where the noonday sun is truly hazardous to skin vitality. Aloe vera is also a natural skin softener.

PABA, an important sunscreening agent by day, will help heal sun-wrecked skin by night.

(*Note:* Apply this serum to the back of your hands as well as to your face. No, this formula won't eradicate sun spots, but it will alleviate dry damage done by the UV rays.)

℞. *If you have older dry skin with noticeable large pores*, add 1 teaspoon sesame oil (see above) and 1 teaspoon ascorbic acid (buy in the drugstore) to base before blending.

Ascorbic acid is another form of vitamin C—a most important vitamin in the formation of collagen, the protein of which skin is made. Here it is serving another function: Its acidity acts as an astringent, or temporary pore tightener.

℞. *If your skin is plagued by under-the-skin bumps*, add 1 teaspoon sesame oil (see above), 1 teaspoon ascorbic acid, and 1 aspirin tablet to the base before blending.

Aspirin contains salicylic acid, a powerful skin-peeling acid used in acne treatment. Dissolved in this formula, it becomes an excellent mild keratolytic (i.e., skin-peeling) agent, helping to make those tiny bumps surface for treatment. Under-the-skin breakout is the dry-skinned woman's form of Messy Skin Syndrome.

℞. *If you have real combination skin, oily in T-zone, very dry on cheeks*, add 1 teaspoon safflower oil and 2 tablespoons vodka to base before blending.

Safflower oil is a lightweight, highly unsaturated oil that will penetrate the skin. Because it is not heavy, it is good for skin that is not completely dry.

Vodka in the mouth ages you; vodka on the skin is a youth tonic. The high-proof alcohol will serve as an excellent toner.

(*Note:* If your skin is mildly oily in the T-zone, use this serum over your entire face; if it is very T-oily, skip the forehead and nose. If you're over 30, the third part of the T, your chin, probably isn't as oily as you think: Serum the chin, too.)

℞. *If your skin type is slightly dry or normal but wrinkled and sagging*, add 1 teaspoon ascorbic acid (see page 61) and 1 egg white to base before blending.

The egg white is pure albumin—pure protein; it works as a natural skin tightener.

℞. *If your dry skin is caused by an overheated/over-air-conditioned environment* (often the curse of women who live in apartments where the landlord controls the thermostat), add 1 teaspoon glycerine to base before blending.

This fatty by-product of soap production is an important water-soluble emollient. Besides softening skin, it also serves as a humectant: Glycerine draws moisture (i.e., water) from the atmosphere to your skin and keeps your skin's own water supply from evaporating into the dry air.

℞. *If your late nights show up as "tired" dry skin*, add 50 mg of vitamin B_2 (riboflavin) to base before blending.

B_2 helps keep the skin from becoming rough and cracked. Bonus: It helps fight the tiny crevices that can form above upper lip. As one of the B family, riboflavin also has a tranquilizing effect.

℞. *If your life style produces lots of stress and tension*, the result is often dry, aggravated skin. Add 50 mg vitamin B_2 (riboflavin) and 50 mg vitamin B_6 (pyridoxine) to base before blending.

B_6, another of the stress-fighting B family of vitamins, also fights eczema and other skin breakouts that may be associated with tension.

℞. *If you never get any physical exercise*, your lethargic dry skin will benefit from the following added to your base before blending: 50 mg vitamin B_2 (see above), 50 mg vitamin B_6 (see above), 100 mg vitamin B_3 (niacin), and 1 tablet inositol.

Vitamin B_3 (niacin) is an important enzyme energizer, and inositol is a "provitamin," meaning that inositol is actually a synergist which helps make other vitamins work together efficiently.

You also need a good workout. Exercise not only keeps your body in shape, it keeps skin glowing. You can follow a carefully tailored skin-care regimen, but if the only physical effort you indulge in is patting on your serum, your skin will never look terrific. That's why you must move your body to see skin improvement. Exercise brings oxygen to the skin and helps "sweat out" impurities. Every complexion will benefit by a body that's kept in motion.

℞. *If your dry skin also marks and scars easily*, your base formula must be expanded to include vitamins B_2, B_6, B_3, and inositol (see page 62). You must also add 10,000 IU vitamin A and 400 IU vitamin D to the base before blending.

Vitamin A, the "skin vitamin," is necessary for a soft, smooth, healthy complexion. If you're vitamin A–deficient, expect to have rough, bumpy-looking skin.

Vitamin D is produced naturally by the effect of sunshine on your skin. Yes, D is important, but get it through fortified milk and vitamins, not by baking in the sun. (Re internal vitamin usage: A and D are both fat-soluble —which means they're stored in the body—so there is a danger of overdose if you ingest too much. Stick with the recommended daily allowances found in your multivitamin supplement, or talk with your doctor before upping your *internal* intake of A and D.)

Vitamins A and D are often combined commercially in ointment form to treat bruised, marked, or scarred skin.

OILY SKIN SLEEP SERUMS: THE "SUPER SIX" BASE

If you have oily skin, your precious brown bottle will be filled with the following six basics, which you will combine according to the formula following this descriptive listing:

▫ *Bubbly Mineral Water* (Perrier, Poland Spring, Saratoga—there are many available). Every night you will "take the cure"—that's what millions of Europeans do each year when they visit the *bäd* (or bath) for some R & R—Restoration and Rejuvenation. Scientific investigations have shown that mineral water is actually absorbed by the skin. Besides containing good-for-your-complexion carbonic acid, these waters also hold traces of other important minerals that will help keep connective tissue healthy. While it may be impractical to bathe your *body* in mineral water (unless you live near the ocean—sea water is chockfull of the best minerals; it's a veritable mineral treasure trove), you can at least treat your face to some hydrotherapy. (Remember, when it comes to mineral water, *bad* is good!) Don't refrigerate your face-serum water; it's more bubbly and effective when applied at room temperature. (You will be using refrigerated water as a face tonic—see Beat-the-Clock Skin-Care System at the end of Part Three; for a discussion of the benefits of *drinking* mineral water, see Chapter 7.)

◻ *Glycerine* is a water-soluble emollient that acts as a humectant: It draws moisture from the air to your skin and helps keep your skin's own water supply locked within the dermis. Remember, even though you have oil-rich skin, your complexion may be water-poor, so you could be dehydrated. Glycerine will help.

◻ *Gelatin*—an easy-to-find (check your supermarket) and easy-to-prepare source of collagen protein.

◻ *Seaweed or Kelp*—a natural thickener high in mineral content and collagen-building vitamin C (see pages 61, 65).

◻ *Multiple Vitamin Tablet*—for multiple nutritional benefits.

◻ *Vitamin C Tablet*—the acid in the C will act as a mild astringent; C also helps build collagen.

Formula for "Super Six" Base

1.	Bubbly Mineral Water	½ cup
2.	Glycerine	1 teaspoon
3.	Unflavored Gelatin Preparation	½ cup
4.	Seaweed or Kelp	1 teaspoon
5.	Multiple Vitamin	1 tablet
6.	Vitamin C, 100 mg	1 tablet

To make, put first two ingredients in blender. To prepare gelatin: Dissolve 1 tablespoon gelatin in ¼ cup cold water; add ¾ cup boiling water to it. Allow to cool to body temperature and add ½ cup of the mix to blender (reserve remainder for use when preparing another oily skin serum). Add remaining ingredients.

The above base is an ℞ in itself *if you have blemish-free oily skin*. It's designed to help any "still oily" woman over the age of 25. If you have a more complicated oily skin problem, consult the ℞s and additives that follow.

℞. *If you have mature oily skin with breakouts* (*Messy Skin Syndrome*), add 2 tablespoons vodka to the basic brew before blending.

If some people we know consumed vodka externally instead of drinking it, perhaps their faces wouldn't resemble boiled potatoes! Vodka will act as an astringent, helping reduce problem-causing excess oil that collects on the skin's surface.

℞. *If your oily skin is accompanied by very large pores*, add 1 teaspoon ascorbic acid to base before blending.

Ascorbic acid, another form of vitamin C, is available in your drugstore. C is an important vitamin in the formation of collagen, the protein of which skin is made. Here, it is serving a dual purpose: Its acidity acts as an astringent, inducing temporary pore tightening. C will also draw off excess surface-clogging oils.

℞. *If you have typical problem skin, oily with small bumpy deposits; wrinkles under eyes and around mouth/nose*, add 1 teaspoon ascorbic acid and 1 aspirin to base before blending.

Aspirin contains salicylic acid, a powerful skin-peeling acid used in acne treatment. Dissolved in this formula, it becomes an excellent mild keratolytic (i.e., skin-peeling) agent, helping to peel the roof off those small oil-clogged bumps so they can surface for treatment.

℞. *If your oily skin is also lined and sagging*, add 1 teaspoon ascorbic acid (see above) and ¼ teaspoon alum to basic brew before blending.

Alum, an aluminum salt (find it in the drugstore) with astringent properties, acts as a temporary pore tightener. It will also hide fine lines and give sagging skin a taut, firm feel.

℞. *If your oily skin needs fast reviving* (after an occasional up-all-night, no-sleep-the-next-day), add 50 mg vitamin B_2 (riboflavin) to base before blending.

B_2 will help keep skin from cracking and fight excess skin oiliness. As one of the B-complex vitamins, riboflavin has a tranquilizing effect.

℞. *If you're a poor sleeper and have chronic tired-looking, lifeless skin*, add 50 mg B_2 (see above) and 1 teaspoon tricalcium phosphate to base before blending.

Tricalcium phosphate (buy in pharmacy) is a natural, soothing tranquilizer also found in milk.

℞. *If you've suffered a traumatic emotional shock and your skin is showing the results*, add 100 IU vitamin E to base before blending.

This is the one exception to the E-is-not-for-oily-skins rule I quoted earlier. If you're going through a traumatic period, and your skin is responding by wrinkling and itching rather than breaking out, the addition of E over a short time span should prove extremely helpful.

℞. *If you're under stress and anxiety and your skin is breaking out*, add

50 mg vitamin B₂ (see page 65) and 50 mg vitamin B₆ (pyridoxine) to base before blending.

B₆ is an important stress-fighting vitamin that also fights eczema, blackheads, and other skin breakouts that may be tension-related.

℞. *If you never have time for exercise, you have lethargic, oily skin.* Add 50 mg B₂ (see page 65), 50 mg B₆ (see page 62) 100 mg B₃ (niacin), and 1 inositol tablet to the base before blending.

B₃, or niacin, is an enzyme energizer that's also useful in fighting skin problems that may appear if your skin never gets a chance to let off trapped sebum via a good workout. Exercise helps skin all over your body and face work up a good sweat and "sweat out" impurities. Your complexion will never get that healthy glow if you don't put your body in motion.

You also need inositol, which isn't exactly a vitamin. As discussed, it helps other vitamins do their job. (See page 62.)

℞. *If your oily skin marks and scars easily*, add 50 mg B₂ (see page 65), 50 mg B₆ (see above), 100 mg B₃, and 1 inositol tablet (see above), as well as 10,000 IU vitamin A and 400 IU vitamin D to base before blending.

Vitamin A, the skin vitamin, is vital for a soft, smooth, and healthy complexion. If you're A-deficient, expect to have rough, bumpy-looking skin.

Vitamin D is produced naturally by the effect of sunshine on your skin. Get it through fortified milk or vitamin supplements, not by baking in the sun.

VITAMINS: THE INTERNAL MIX

So far I've spoken about using vitamins in skin serums. What about *taking* vitamins? There are certain basics for both good health and beauty that I believe should be part of your daily intake. They include:

One multivitamin-mineral combination supplement. Compare labels and buy the formula that offers you more. Take your vitamin as a "chaser" to a meal. Vitamins work best in conjunction with food, so down your supplements after your meals.

The B-complex vitamins. I've mentioned the importance of B₂ (riboflavin), B₃ (niacin), B₆ (pyridoxine), inositol, PABA. These are just some of the B-for-Beauty vitamins. If you want to avoid getting a "complex" yourself, you'll take a nerve-calming, stress-curbing B pill daily. B is also important in the control of skin breakouts, the development of red blood cells, and the promotion of skin suppleness and health. How much B₂ should you ingest? Or niacin? Or inositol? Unless you're friendly with a health guru or nutritionist, it's dangerous to use these supplements individually and dose yourself on a daily basis. (If you are undergoing a period of stress, you may want to up your intake of various Bs on a *temporary* basis—see page 70.)

No, they're not fat-soluble, so they won't build up in your system . . . but if you take too much of one B regularly, you may unknowingly increase your need for one of the companion Bs. Let the vitamin makers take the guess-work out of your everyday B-boost: Buy all the Bs in one tablet or capsule labeled "B Complex"—for energy, tranquility, and skin health (more about the Bs and hair health later).

If you equate *vitamin C* with the common cold, it's time to expand your definition. Let C stand for collagen production. Collagen is the protein healthy skin is made of, and you have to do your part in maintaining a good collagen supply by using collagen-rich face treatment creams and insuring an adequate intake of vitamin C, either via food (citrus fruits, peppers, cauli-flower, and tomatoes are good C sources) or via vitamins. C also helps fight broken capillaries and stress. As mentioned earlier, smokers need a greater C intake (they lose 25 mg per cigarette); so do drinkers (if you're a moderate or more drinker, you need that important B complex, too). You should be taking a 100 mg C supplement daily.

If you're under a doctor's care for any reason, or if you're pregnant or taking the Pill, be sure to check out any change in vitamin intake with your physician. If you're interested in learning more about vitamins and nutrition, read Adelle Davis's books. Adelle was (and is) to health buffs what Agatha was (is) to mystery fans.

CHAPTER 5

🏵🏵🏵

Round-the-World
10-Years-Off Roundup

While Prescription Sleep Serums inspired by legendary Alpine sleep cures and modern European know-how should be part of your beauty regimen, no guided youth and beauty tour would be complete without introducing you to additional important beauty treatments adapted from other times, other cultures. What follows is a potpourri of excellent treatments for your face and body.

FROM THE BALKANS: THE PLASMA PACK FACIAL AND DRACULA ENERGIZING DRINK

Good skin depends on many factors, as I've stated, not the least of which is a healthy blood supply to the face.

European women have been aware of this fact for centuries. Next to mineral water, used both internally and externally, beauties "over there" rejuvenate their skins via what I call the "Transylvanian Transfusion," a plasma-rich facial and accompanying nutritious drink. These wonderful skin boosters and restoratives first emerged in the Balkan cradle of beauty culture.

History. Blood as a beauty source has taken on a bad press ever since the Dracula legend was revived by the novel of the same name and cape-clad Bela Lugosi flew fang-first across the wide screen into our collective fantasies.

The most famous real-life vampire was certainly no lady, but she was a woman. In the 17th century, Countess Bathory of Vienna murdered several hundred young virgins and drank their blood; she felt virginal hemoglobin was one terrific youth tonic. Madame Bathory didn't live long enough to prove her theory, however—she died three years after being imprisoned for her crimes.

Am I suggesting that you don a black cape and haunt the local blood bank between midnight and sunrise? Not quite! Nor do I suggest you try to assemble a brace of young virgins (they're becoming somewhat of an endangered species).

But I *do* recommend that you give yourself my plasma facial, a true power pack for your skin, rich in iron and blood-forming vitamins. You should also feed your face internally with the B-rich nutritional drink that follows. The internal and external benefits of this mini-plasma program will give your complexion a tremendous boost. And there's nothing immoral or illegal about it.

Too bad Countess B. didn't have our modern scientific know-how. In my professional serum collection, sold in department stores, we combine bovine (cow) plasma, the clear, noncellular fluid portion of the blood, with bovine albumin, a blood protein also derived from cattle. The chemical nature of blood serum is closely related to the chemical nature of skin; the affinity between the two can have a beneficial effect on your complexion.

Your at-home Plasma Pack Facial will be made in your blender in much the same way as your night serums. Ingredients include:

- *Soybean Oil*—a lightweight, polyunsaturated oil that's naturally good for your skin.
- *Vitamin B Complex*—besides having a tranquilizing effect, the B vitamins are most important in the formation of red blood cells. While B stands for beauty, it also stands for blood!
- *Vitamin B$_{12}$*—an important B-vite component. It not only helps red blood cells form; it regenerates the red cells you've got.
- *Liver*—one of the richest sources of the B vitamins, iron, and vitamin C (important in collagen formation). I smash raw liver into my own transfusion; some prefer to omit the raw and stick with desiccated (dried) liver, which you can buy in tablet form in your pharmacy or health food store.
- *Iron*—carries oxygen in the blood to the tissues; most important for good skin color.
- *Sesame Oil*—25 percent vitamin E; your skin will drink it up.
- *Lecithin*—a natural emulsifier rich in B vitamins and vitamin E; it will keep your "transfusion" well blended.
- *Cod Liver Oil*—rich in the skin vitamins, A and D.
- *Unflavored Gelatin Preparation*—a collagen source.

The Plasma Pack Facial

1. Soybean Oil	½ cup
2. Vitamin B Complex	1 tablet
3. Vitamin B$_{12}$	1 capsule
4. Desiccated Liver	2 tablets
or	
5. Raw Liver (optional)	2-inch cube
6. Iron	1 tablet
7. Sesame Oil	1 tablespoon
8. Lecithin	2 tablespoons
9. Cod Liver Oil	½ tablespoon
10. Unflavored Gelatin Preparation	½ cup

To make, put first nine ingredients in blender. Prepare gelatin as for Prescription Sleep Serums (see page 60).

Mix in blender, leave on face 10 minutes. Rinse with cool water. This pack makes an excellent monthly heavy-duty face treatment.

The "Dracula" Energizing Drink: A Blood-Building Tension-Fighting Beauty Tonic

A pale, wan complexion can be the result of less than vigorous blood circulation, lack of protein, or a sudden surge of stress/tension in your life. This drink is rich in various components of the B complex; it will help build protein, fight stress, and develop healthy red blood cells. It's not meant as a daily tonic; save it for those times when your vitality is at a low ebb, your nerves are unraveling in high gear, and you need the depression-fighting boost a B surplus will give you.

Mix the following in your blender until smooth:

1. ½ cup Cranberry Juice
2. ½ cup bubbly Mineral Water
3. ½ teaspoon Epsom Salts (Magnesium Sulfate)
4. ½ teaspoon Calcium Phosphate
5. 1 tablet Vitamin B$_6$ (25 mg)
6. 1 tablet Pantothenic Acid (50 mg)
7. 1 tablet Vitamin B$_3$ (Niacin, 100 mg)
8. 1 tablet Vitamin C (300 mg)
9. 1 teaspoon Amino Acid Powder
10. 1 Liver Tablet (with Vitamin B$_{12}$) (750 mg Liver + 5 mg Vitamin B$_{12}$)
11. 1 teaspoon Brewer's Yeast Powder
12. 1 tablet Multivitamin

What will the above brew do for you? Consider the following:

Cranberry juice contains quinic acid, which has the ability to help rid the body of dead cells.

Mineral water is a natural source of important minerals your diet may not supply in abundance.

Epsom salts are a readily available source of magnesium sulfate, a prime stress-fighting mineral.

Calcium phosphate also helps ease tension.

Vitamin B$_6$ helps develop healthy red blood cells, fights anemia and skin disorders, and acts as a nerve "tranquilizer."

Pantothenic acid is another B component found in many commercially available stress formulations; it is often called the "stress vitamin." Liver and brewer's yeast are excellent natural sources of fatigue-fighting pantothenic acid.

B$_3$ (*niacin or niacinamide*) is an enzyme energizer (it helps various complicated body functions function properly!) and tension fighter (there is some evidence that it also helps control schizophrenia—hopefully you're not that depressed). As a B-for-Blood vitamin, niacin also helps build red cells and fight anemia.

Vitamin C, as I mentioned, is essential for collagen formation. Among its many additional uses, it fights stress. Along with pantothenic acid, C is a component in commercially sold stress tablets.

Amino acids are the building blocks of protein and blood.

Liver is rich in iron and other minerals and vitamins. Consider liver essential for energy. (Desiccated liver is a good substitute for cooked liver if you refuse to make the latter part of your weekly diet.) B$_{12}$ is often called the "pep vitamin"; it helps prevent anemia and fatigue and promotes an energetic feeling as well as healthy red blood cells.

Brewer's yeast is rich in B vitamins, protein, minerals. It is an excellent fatigue-fighting food.

A multivitamin tablet is for multiple, broad-based nutritional benefits.

The above energy-giving, tension-fighting, B-for-Blood tonic should have been quaffed by the legendary vampires. Their thirst for corpuscles would have been nutritiously sated by this vitamin-powered beauty-promoting boost to their blood supply. (But then, what would have become of Bela Lugosi?)

FROM SWEDEN:
SHOCK THERAPY: THE SWEDISH FREEZE

In Scandinavia, cold water therapy is highly respected and an ice-cold shower is part of many stay-young programs because it promotes greater oxygen intake in the cells and helps increase blood circulation.

You can use cold water on your face as an instant pick-me-up before a public appearance or a big evening out, when you want to tighten your skin and temporarily soften wrinkles. But a few desultory splashes of H_2O aren't enough. You need to take advantage of the Swedish Freeze, prepared-in-advance cold shock therapy designed to wake up your tired, sagging face.

Here's what you do: Take a plastic ice cube tray you'll set aside for this purpose and fill with a solution of ½ mineral water, ½ astringent (or freshener) and two pinches of alum. Fill each cube ½ full (the water will expand as it freezes) with the above mixture and angle a tongue depressor into each cube. You will have to remove one ice tray if you put in ice compartment of your refrigerator, or freeze in larger freezer compartment.

When you want to wake your face, pop out one "serving" and, using the stick as a handle, rub over your entire face till you feel it tingle. Then press the ice treatment over noticeable lines (this skin pressing is a variation of the cold iron treatment I use in my salons). You're actually softening the appearance of wrinkles by tightening the skin surrounding them; this will help give your complexion a firm, fresh texture.

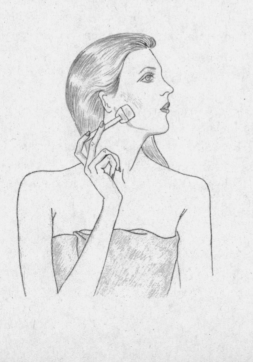

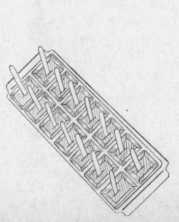

FROM ANCIENT EGYPT:
THE NEFERTITI FACE-AND-BREAST LIFT

The Egyptians of thousands of years ago were even more ambitious than the most devoted of today's youth clinicians. Not only were they interested in keeping *living* faces and bodies young looking (witness Cleopatra and her milk baths, essential oil treatments, and henna-based cosmetics); they also devised an elaborate embalming process to keep the body firm and intact for the long voyage to *eternity*. (The shape and temperature of the pyramids themselves were allegedly designed to help preserve the body in its earthly state for generations.)

While the study of afterlife "pyramid power" is best left to Tutmaniacs and knowledgeable high priestesses, I want to give you a treatment that works wonders in *preserving the skin of the living*.

Ancient Skin Preservation (A.S.P.) Moisturizing Formula

1. Anhydrous Lanolin   ½ cup (available at drugstores)
2. Safflower Oil   ½ cup (available at health food stores or supermarkets)
3. Vitamin A, 10,000 IU   1 tablet
4. Vitamin E, 100 IU   1 capsule
5. Vitamin D, 400 IU   1 tablet

To make, melt anhydrous lanolin and mix with safflower oil. Cool, add vitamins, and blend well.

"Mummified" Gauze Wrap Solution

1. Mineral Water   1 cup
2. Liquid Pectin   1 ounce
3. Lemon Juice   1 teaspoon
    (reconstituted or fresh)
4. Vitamin C, 100 mg   1 tablet
5. Alum   1 teaspoon

Liquid pectin (Certo is a widely available brand) is used in preserving jams and jellies and can be found in your supermarket. This gauze solution is acidic (thanks to lemon juice, vitamin C/ascorbic acid)—it will firm and tighten your skin and temporarily refine pores.

To prepare, mix ingredients well.

Now that you have your formula and solution, you're ready to begin the two-step treatment. Step #1 is a moisturizing massage, step #2 a tightening wrap.

Step #1: Ancient Skin Preservation Massage

Cover hair with towel. Massage moisturizing formula into face, throat, and breasts in the following manner.

Face: Start with fingertips of both hands poised on chin. Massage liberally into center of face with upward motion, avoiding eye area. Place fingertips in center of forehead, massage outward and along border of face.

Throat: With entire fingers flattened against neck, start at collarbone and work into skin of throat up to chin with long, upward, sweeping strokes.

Breasts: Massage into breasts, using fingers in circular motion. Make sure you coat sides and beneath breasts with formula.

Leave in place.

Step #2: Mummified Face and Breast Wrap

Cut three strips of 2-inch-wide gauze to cover face and throat as illustrated, plus additional lengths of gauze to wrap breasts, and dip all strips in solution. (The solution stiffens the gauze, molding it to your skin.)

Gently squeeze out excess solution and press gauze over the A.S.P. formula, which should still be in place on skin, in the following pattern:

Mold first piece of gauze on neck.

Mold second strip over chin and cheek area.

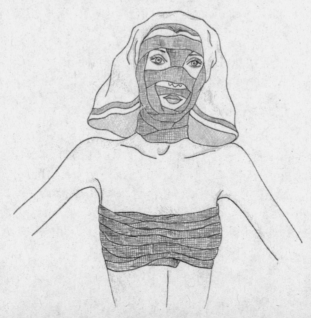

Mold third strip on forehead and pull into place over entire upper portion of face. Cover the nose, but leave nostrils and mouth exposed. Mold mouth and nose areas into place, and pull the ends of each strip upward until they have conformed to the contours of the face.

Wrap breasts by pulling longer gauze strips firmly, starting high along side of left breast; extend same strip under breasts and up along side of right breast, so breasts are lifted. Mold additional gauze across front of breasts. Rinse fingers (which are probably sticky from solution) under tap water.

Lie down and rest for 10 minutes, letting the gauze harden, or mummify.

Unmold gauze, dampen washcloth with tepid water, and gently wipe away residue.

As noted, your skin will have received deep moisturization from the formula and temporary tightening from the wrap.

FROM THE ORIENT:
THE ARPEL ACUPRESSURE ADAPTATION,
EAST-MEETS-WEST FACE-LIFT

Historians tell us that the Chinese invented gunpowder, tea, and noodles. Important, yes, but from a beauty standpoint the number one import on the Oriental hit parade is acupressure, the laying-on-of-hands art that can help restore the bloom to your suddenly-looking-venerable cheeks (it's fine for ancient students of Confucius to look wise and venerable—not so terrific if you look 30-going-on-50).

Acupressure is really do-it-yourself acupuncture, or acupuncture without needles. So let me say a few words about acupuncture first.

The Chinese believe that to insure bodily health, youth, and vigor, the balance of yin (female) and yang (male) elements that reside in each of us must be maintained. They further believe that when one is ill, the energy inside the body is blocked, and the yin/yang harmony is destroyed. To restore the harmony and alleviate pain and sickness, needles are inserted in one or more (usually many more) of the specially designated 600-odd acupuncture points to get the energy once again flowing properly. If you have ever seen an acupuncture chart, you have noticed it is filled with a dizzying maze of hundreds of intersecting lines and points.

Needless to say, this Oriental art is practically inscrutable to most Westerners and the correct application of the needles (used for everything from arthritis abatement to a migraine cure) is *not* a do-it-yourself job, unless you want to turn yourself into a walking pincushion.

Face-Lift-by-Acupuncture

The newest acupuncture application, one that has caused a sensation in New York, has nothing to do with illness; it is the use of needle therapy for face-lifts. Many clients (not to mention practitioners) swear by its effectiveness, with the most satisfied reporting lifted jowls, disappearing neck lines, improved muscle tone, softened wrinkles. It's a many-session procedure in which fine needles may be applied to the calves and hands as well as the face (it all depends on where the points for face muscle tone and circulation are located); it's also less traumatic (and cheaper), though less overnight dramatic, than a conventional under-the-knife face-lift.

The Arpel Acupressure Adaptation

While it takes a trained acupuncturist to perform a face-lift by needles (and a pioneering sort of woman to submit to the multiple needle treatment), you can improve facial muscle tone yourself and prevent some premature lining and bagging by combining the Eastern tradition of *acupressure* (the acupuncture derivative, substituting careful placement of the thumbs, fingers, and hands for the needles) with the Western system of toning face muscles through exercise.

The A.A.A. system (my apologies to the American Automobile Association) for face improvement takes just *5 minutes a day, 3 days a week*. But I'm going to ask you to work just a few minutes more. I don't believe the face should be exercised or manually manipulated in any way unless a massage ointment is applied first. The proper ointment will help your fingers glide over your skin, prevent the heavy-handed from tugging and pulling delicate tissue. The following acupressure exercise serum is for all skin types and makes enough for your 3-times-weekly routine.

Ginseng Acupressure Exercise Serum

1. Bubbly Mineral Water   ½ cup
2. Glycerine   1 teaspoon
3. Unflavored Gelatin Preparation   ½ cup
4. Seaweed or Kelp   1 teaspoon
5. Multiple Vitamin   1 tablet
6. Vitamin C, 100 mg   1 tablet
7. Ginseng, 2-inch root   1 tablespoon ginseng root, grated, ginseng powder, or crushed ginseng tablets

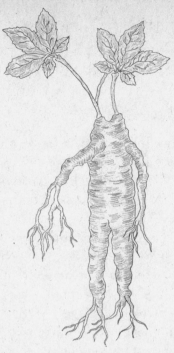

The special ingredient added to this serum is ginseng, also called the "man-root" because it is indeed shaped like a man. Ginseng has been an important part of Oriental folk medicine for some 5,000 years. Although high-quality ginseng is extraordinarily expensive, Koreans and Chinese of the most limited means still use their savings to purchase the root. The reason: It is believed to have rejuvenating properties. For our purposes, I have included ginseng for its ability to rebuild body tissues and promote normal cell growth. Buy the root in Oriental food stores and scrape off the equivalent of one tablespoon into your blender. (You may find it more convenient to use the powder or tablet form, available in health food stores.)

To make, put first two ingredients in blender. Prepare gelatin as for Prescription Sleep Serums (see page 60). Add remaining ingredients, blend well.

Ginseng Tea

While you're aboard my youth clinic tour of the Orient, I want to introduce you to ginseng tea (available in health food stores). A cup in the morning should replace your traditional coffee break if you tire easily. Ginseng is a favorite "tonic" for those who complain of overwhelming fatigue; it may also be a stress abater. Some swear the man-shaped ginseng root, considered the most yang (masculine) of herbs, is a powerful aphrodisiac. While I can't swear to the truth of the yang-producing/impotence-fighting quality of the herb, the man-root has been reported to help *women* fight menstrual cramps and curb the hot flashes often associated with menopause.

East-Meets-West Face-Lift: Preliminaries

My East-Meets-West Face-Lift combines the tension-easing and circulation-boosting benefits of acupressure with the muscle-toning movements of our own culture. This is a routine that I have followed with visible improvement on my own skin. Try it yourself and you'll be doing your present and future face a great service.

Understand that the "pressure" part of the routine is important, because by taming tension and improving circulation to the face you are working not only to prevent new lines, but to soften wrinkles that have already appeared. Good circulation also promotes a healthy glow, a sign of young skin. (A wan, colorless complexion does *not* suggest feminine fragility. Rather, it indicates a complexion whose bloom has long since faded from the rose.)

The pressure you'll apply in most of these routines should be moderate: not featherweight, but not so heavy that you leave fingerprints on your skin. Exceptions will be noted.

Pick and Choose

You won't necessarily be doing all of the exercises. Just follow the ones geared to your own trouble spots, performing your chosen series 3 times a week. You will probably need a 3-session intensive, extended training period to get the finger motions down properly. But once you've mastered the movements, you will be able to zip right through the regimen that follows in about 5 minutes. If you can spare those 5 minutes, do practice the entire Arpel Acupressure Adaptation and you will be taking a front-line stand in the fight against lines and wrinkles.

Suggestion: Perform face-lift while looking in the mirror when possible, so you can make sure facial muscles are completely relaxed during each set.

The Forehead: to Soften Horizontal Lines

Apply Ginseng Acupressure Exercise Serum to forehead.

Place 4 fingers (arched) of both hands in center of forehead. Press for 5 seconds. Gradually separate fingertips at ½-inch intervals, repeating 5-second press until fingers of each hand reach the temples.

Take arched fingers, turn the other way, and rest on eyebrows. Press

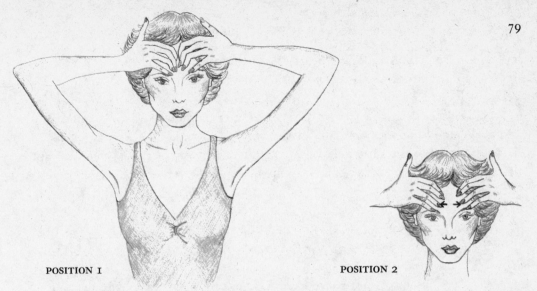

POSITION I   POSITION 2

for 5 seconds and move up forehead to hairline in ½-inch intervals, repeating 5-second press at each interval.

Return fingers to original position. Apply more serum if necessary. Stroke across forehead from center to temples 15 times. Your forehead should now feel completely relaxed; your horizontal lines are softening.

Exactly *how* does acupressure work? While Western scientists can't give a definitive answer, they admit that, like its parent, acupuncture, this Oriental technique does produce results. If you can suspend your disbelief of anything that doesn't submit to a technical equation, and let your face speak for itself, you shouldn't care whether you're practicing an art, science, or 17th-century witchcraft.

The Forehead: to Soften Vertical Scowl Lines

With one thumb on top of the other, press area located between your brows—known in India as the "third eye." (While the names change, many

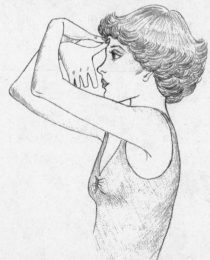

cultures have come to the independent conclusion that the same parts of the face and body are keys to inner health.) Maintain moderate pressure for 10 seconds. Repeat 3 times.

How long will it be before you see results? While it was all-American Ralph Waldo Emerson who said "patience and fortitude in all things," surely he was related to the Oriental sages. The effect is *cumulative*—if you keep at it for at least 3 months, your newly acquired Western patience will be rewarded.

The Eyes: to Ease Strain, Soften Crow's-Feet and Squint Lines

Apply Ginseng Acupressure Exercise Serum to eyelids and under eyes.

Cover closed eyes with 3 middle fingers in horizontal position. Apply slight pressure. Hold in place for 10 seconds, without moving eyelid skin. Repeat once. Crow's-feet, undereyes, and upper lids should be completely covered. This relaxes the eye area. (Position 1 below)

Put same 3 fingers perpendicular to eyes on bone under brow. Rest thumbs under cheekbone for balance. Stroke from inner to outer eyelid and across crow's-feet. (Position 2 below)

As you reach lower lid, use balls of fingers to create light pressure movements. Press, don't stroke, lower lid area. Circle eye with this combination stroke/pat routine 5 times.

Romantic Western poets believe the eye is the window of the soul. Pragmatic Eastern doctors feel the eye is the mirror of the internal organs. Bright, healthy-looking eyes surrounded by soft, smooth skin not only make you look young and alert, they also indicate your yin and yang are in harmony and energy is coursing through your body.

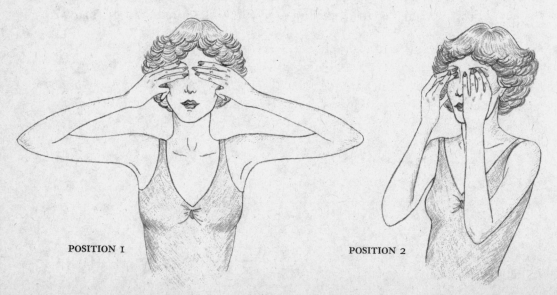

POSITION 1   POSITION 2

The Cheeks: to Fill Out and Firm Cheek Contour

Apply Ginseng Acupressure Exercise Serum to cheeks.

Hook thumbs lightly under chin and press index finger on a line 1 ½ inches below iris. Hold pressure 5 seconds; repeat 3 times.

Place same index finger on outer cheekbones, repeat procedure.

With thumbs still in place, slide index finger 10 times across the two pressure points just manipulated and continue in outward arc to *top* of the ear.

Puff out left cheek with air; hold 3 seconds. Let collapse. Repeat 3 times, then follow same routine on right cheek.

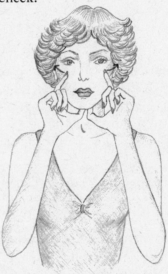

Mouth Area: to Fill Out Nose-to-Mouth Lines,
Offer Some Help for Wrinkles above Upper Lip

Apply Ginseng Acupressure Exercise Serum around mouth.

With mouth in relaxed, slightly open position, place index finger in groove above center of upper lip; place thumb in chin groove under lower lip. Press moderately for 5 seconds. Repeat once.

Place thumb and index finger just to the side of mouth corners. Hold 5 seconds; repeat once.

Stretch upper lip to cover upper teeth. At the same time, cover lower teeth with lower lip. Hold 5 seconds; repeat 3 times.

To correct droopy mouth corners, which can age you prematurely by giving you a forlorn appearance, the best exercise is to smile—really smile—

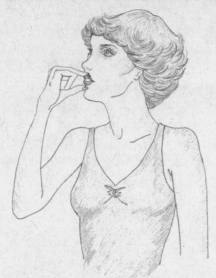

with your mouth closed. Exaggeratedly curl your lips upward. Smile and laugh whenever you can for a happy, young look. But check your mirror. It isn't necessary to wrinkle your eyes when you smile. It takes practice, but you can laugh with your mouth only.

Chin, Throat: to Prevent and Alleviate Double Chin, Less-than-Taut Throat

Apply Ginseng Acupressure Exercise Serum to chin and throat.

With chin slightly elevated, place tips of thumbs together in hollow behind jawbone. Press firmly for 10 seconds, release; repeat 3 times.

With chin pointing toward ceiling, mouth lightly closed, stick out lower jaw as far as you can. Feel your neck tendons stretch. Hold for 10 seconds; repeat 3 times.

With chin pointing toward ceiling and neck stretched taut, circle your collarbone with both hands and smooth neck with long upward strokes from collarbone to chin. Repeat 5 times. Make sure your neck is well serumed.

FROM THE U.S.A.:
THE SNIP-AND-TUCK WRINKLE TRAINER

While it may take great courage to divest yourself of a frown-causing man or job, it takes just a small investment in time and effort to smooth the lines that tension and poor facial habits combine to cause.

What you have to do is put your face in "training." You train your lines to flatten, either while you sleep, or during the day when you're home alone. All you need in the way of equipment is gummed labels (available in any stationery store), which you'll cut into a convenient diamond, half-butterfly, or circular shape (whichever will best cover your wrinkle). Now, here's how to use:

Cleanse, rinse, and dry skin thoroughly.

Rub the wrinkles against the grain (horizontally for vertical scowl lines; vertically for across-the-brow furrows) to stimulate circulation (till you feel slight friction).

Moisten gummed label with warm water and press in place (don't tug on your skin) over line you want to soften.

To fight expression lining, try to keep in place a half hour a day, 3 times a week.

If you're under stress, beef up your training by eliminating your serum one night a week and sleeping with your wrinkle trainer in place for an 8-hour treatment.

To remove, moisten label and lift gently off skin (don't tear—it's not a Band-Aid). Splash face 10 times with warm (not hot) water and moisturize.

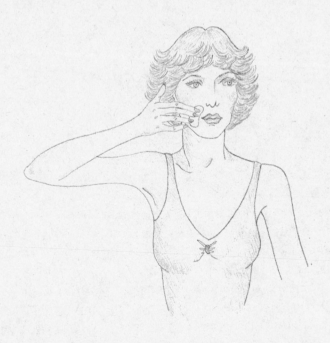

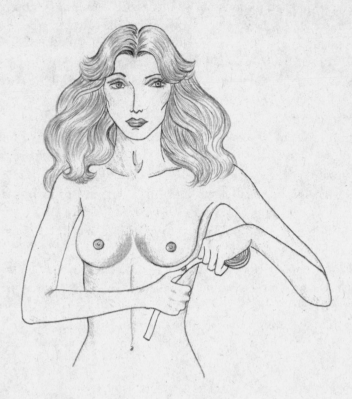

FROM THE U.S.A.:
THE MODELS' SUBTRACT-10-YEARS
BREAST-LIFT

Our own culture specializes in fast food, fast cars, fast action . . . why not a fast body change? If you're wearing a dress that requires the no-bra look but your bosom is on the small size and you're no longer as firm as you'd like to be, all you need is a roll of Scotch tape and the following instructions:

Tear off one piece of ½-inch tape that's long enough to cup your breasts from under one arm, down beneath the breasts where underwire from bra would rest, up, and under the other arm. Use one arm to cradle your breasts and push them together. Your fingers will meet the fingers of your other hand, and together they will start to secure the tape to your skin. Keep your breasts together as you tape, and you'll be creating instant cleavage. (It's easier to do than to describe. In this case, a picture really is worth a thousand words—just follow the illustration.)

Models and actresses have been using this tape trick for years; they also highlight their newly discovered cleavage with a bit of blusher.

CHAPTER 6

❦❦❦

The Beat-the-Clock
Skin-Care System

Now that you have "attended" the serum and round-the-world workshops and learned how to fight the big six premature agers by absorbing the information in Part Two, you're ready to line up your treatment products and set up your own anti-aging skin-care regimen.

The information in this chapter is divided into treatment routines geared to specific skin types. Turn to the condition that describes your skin, and you'll have at your fingertips a practical 10-years-off skin-saving program.

Note: The Arpel Acupressure Adaptation is listed under everyone's skin type because all skins will benefit. The other round-the-world treatments are not included under the various skin-type headings. Rather, you will add these to your personalized regimen as your skin (and your schedule) permits.

DRY SKIN, MINIMUM WRINKLES

Daily P.M.

1. Make-up melt: cold cream. Leave on 60 seconds; remove with wet, warm washcloth, not tissue.
2. Cleanse: Use foaming soap replacement liquid cleanser. Make sure

face is thoroughly wet before applying. Work into lather, spread on with fingertips. Remove by splashing at least 10 times with tepid water.

3. Close eyes and hydrate with plant sprayer filled with mix of ½ mineral water, ½ freshener.

4. Apply eye oil on both upper and lower lids. Pat gently into place with fingertip. Never rub delicate eye-area skin.

5. With skin still damp, apply Prescription Sleep Serum geared to your specific skin problem. Let skin absorb it before you slide into bed (so you won't slide out again).

Daily A.M.

1. Cleanse as in step 2, above.

2. With skin slightly damp, apply nonalcoholic freshener using saturated cotton ball.

3. Apply daytime face treatment cream with fingers. Let sink in.

4. Follow with moisturizer on face and throat.

5. Make up (see Part Six).

Plus Treatments

Add these extras to your skin-care schedule as directed for stay-young skin benefits.

1. Slough with commercial peel-off and fingertips once a week.

2. Arpel Acupressure Adaptation (A.A.A.) 3 times a week.

3. Moisturizing gel mask once a week.

DRY SKIN, NOTICEABLE WRINKLES

Daily P.M.

1. Make-up melt: cold cream. Apply as per instructions in step 1, page 85.

2. Cleanse: cream-based cleanser containing emollients such as lanolin. Remove with wet, warm washcloth held against face to dissolve cleanser. Rinse at least 10 times with tepid water.

3. Hydrate with combination ½ mineral water, ½ freshener. Spray, spray, spray.

4. Pat on eye oil as per step 4 of treatment routine for dry skin with minimum wrinkles, above.

5. Apply your Prescription Sleep Serum generously. Make sure you cover your throat as well as your face.

Daily A.M.

1. Cleanse: Splash with warm (not hot) water 10 times; cool water 10 times. No additional cleanser necessary.
2. Sweep nonalcoholic freshener over face with cotton ball.
3. Massage daytime nourishing treatment cream into face.
4. Apply throat cream with upward strokes.
5. Smooth on moisturizer before applying make-up.

Plus Treatments

Add these extras to your skin-care schedule for stay-young skin benefits.
1. Slough once every 14 days—that's about how often skin rejuvenates itself—with abrasive cream-based scrub containing "gritties" like crushed almonds, oatmeal, apricot kernels, pumice.
2. A.A.A. exercise system 3 times a week.
3. Gel mask every 5 days.

OILY SKIN, MINIMUM WRINKLES, SUFFERING FROM MESSY SKIN SYNDROME

Daily P.M.

1. Make-up melt: Lather once with foaming cleanser to dislodge make-up. Remove with wet, hot washcloth. Heat will help unplug pores.
2. Cleanse with abrasive scrub in cream form or soap containing cleansing grains (i.e., pumice, sea kelp, apricot kernels, oatmeal, almonds).
3. Hydrate skin with mix of ½ astringent, ½ bubbly mineral water. Spray face well.
4. Apply eye oil in stick form to reduce chance of oil's sliding onto blemishes.
5. Smooth on Prescription Sleep Serum geared to your skin problem 2 nights out of 3. On third night, sleep bare-faced except for your eye oil. It isn't necessary for you to serum your throat.

Daily A.M.

1. Cleanse with foaming soap replacement liquid (made by many companies).

2. Exception: Use straight astringent for the duration of your skin breakout problem. Apply with saturated cotton balls (change soiled balls frequently), taking care to avoid deepening lines (i.e., horizontal forehead grooves, nose-to-mouth laugh lines).

3. Stroke on eye oil stick, nutritious day cream (look for one that feels nongreasy; try it before you buy it).

4. Apply moisturizing blotting lotion (made by many companies); besides emollients, they contain keratolytic—i.e., peeling—agents.

5. Apply make-up (see Part Six for specific how-tos).

Plus Treatments

Add these extras to your skin-care schedule for stay-young skin benefits.

1. Slough with cleansing grains and Buf-Puf sponge twice a week.

2. Treat face to a 3-minute herbal steam bath twice weekly, on days alternate from sloughing days. (How-tos, page 23.)

3. A.A.A. exercise system 3 times a week.

4. Spearmint-type mask once a week. It absorbs oils, but it's not as strong as the mud variety.

5. Deep-cleanse with mud mask every other week as long as skin is still messy.

OILY SKIN, WRINKLED

Daily P.M.

1. Make-up melt: foaming soap replacement liquid to dislodge make-up.

2. Cleanse: If skin doesn't feel clean enough after above step, lather again. Even though your skin is oily, it is lined, so you don't want to wash daily with anything abrasive.

3. Spray with ½ freshener, ½ mineral water mix.

4. Apply eye oil in stick form; trace noticeable lines on face with eye oil stick, too.

5. Smooth Prescription Sleep Serum generously into skin. If face is lining, so is neck: Make sure you apply serum to throat.

Daily A.M.

1. Wash with foaming soap replacement liquid cleanser.
2. Use nonalcoholic freshener full strength. It will help lift out oils without drying.
3. Apply eye oil stick.
4. Apply collagen-containing day cream.
5. Follow with moisturizing blotting lotion.
6. Make up.

Plus Treatments

Add these extras to your skin-care regimen for stay-young skin benefits.
1. Slough with cleansing grains and soft complexion brush twice weekly.
2. Treat face to a 3-minute herbal steam bath twice weekly, on days alternate from sloughing days. (How-tos, page 23.)
3. A.A.A. exercise system 3 times a week.
4. Look for mask for normal skin that won't dry hard and fast and leave skin taut.

NORMAL SKIN OVER 30, SOME WRINKLING

Daily P.M.

1. Make-up melt: If you wear full make-up, use cold cream. If you wear minimal make-up, a foaming cleanser will suffice.
2. If skin doesn't feel clean after make-up removal, lather again with foaming cleanser and remove by splashing with tepid water till all traces of residue are gone.
3. Spray with refrigerated mineral water for a hydrating pick-me-up. Don't dry skin completely.
4. Apply eye oil.
5. With skin still damp, apply one of the Prescription Sleep Serums that best matches your skin type. While it may not be necessary to apply to throat yet, it soon will be . . . so why not get a head start?

Daily A.M.

1. You've cleansed well the night before? Refresh your face with 10 splashes of warm water, 10 of cool. If you need additional cleansing, lather once with your foaming soap replacement liquid.

2. Tone with a mix of ½ mineral water, ½ freshener or rose water. Apply with cotton balls.

3. Apply eye protection in oil or stick form. (Stick fans, make sure the product you choose glides easily across your skin. If you have to drag it, toss it: It's doing more harm than good.)

4. Apply day cream.

5. Moisturize.

6. Make up.

Plus Treatments

Add these extras to your skin-care regimen for stay-young skin benefits.

1. Slough once a week with honey and almond scrub or commercial peel-off. If you have remnants of an oily T-zone, slough the T more often.

2. A.A.A. exercise system 3 times a week.

3. Gel mask once a week.

4. Clay mask monthly to deep-clean your pores.

NORMAL SKIN OVER 30, HEAVILY LINED AND WRINKLED

Daily P.M.

1. Make-up melt: cold cream. Apply, let sit for 60 seconds. Remove with warm, wet washcloth.

2. Cleanse with emollient-rich cream-based cleanser containing ingredients like lanolin and coconut derivatives for softening and soothing skin. Rinse well with tepid water.

3. Spray face with mineral water.

4. Pat on eye oil. With Q-tip, smooth eye oil into noticeable lines and wrinkles; let sink in.

5. Apply chosen Prescription Sleep Serum to face and throat.

Daily A.M.

1. Wash with water only: 30 splashes warm followed by 10 splashes cool.

2. Spray with mix of ½ mineral water, ½ nonalcoholic freshener.

3. Add nourishing day cream to face and throat.

4. If your heavily lined skin is accompanied by puffiness around eyes, put refrigerated tea bags over closed eyelids and lie down for 5 minutes while waiting for day cream to penetrate.

5. Moisturize.

6. Make up.

Plus Treatments

Add these extras to your skin-care regimen for stay-young skin benefits.

1. To slough, perform a "salabrasion" (check page 33 for how-to) once every 10 days.

2. Gel mask once a week. Have two gel masks on hand and alternate usage. (Skin gets "bored," doesn't respond to same formula if repeated too often.)

3. Cleanse with spearmint-type mask once every 6 weeks.

4. A.A.A. exercise system 3 times a week.

BONUS: CARE OF THE PREGNANT FACE

If your doctor just said, "Congratulations, you're about to be a mother!" you have to alter your skin-care system temporarily because changes in your body's estrogen/progesterone production may show up on your skin. Here's how the hormones operate: During the first five months of pregnancy, the production of natural lubricating skin oils is suppressed by an increased estrogen production, so your skin may look and feel dry. During the latter half of your pregnancy, there's an upswing in progesterone—so your skin may become *oilier*.

To keep your skin supple during the first five months, do the following:

1. Use a mild, nondetergent cleanser; rinse your face in lukewarm or cool water (hot water is dehydrating).

2. Spray with mineral water before going outdoors.

3. Keep a moisturizer in place all day; apply it over a nourishing day cream containing collagen.

4. If you wear foundation, try using a lightweight "whipped" cream instead of a lotion.

5. At bedtime, make and massage in the "Magnificent Eight" Base Prescription Sleep Serum. (See Chapter 4.)

During the last four months of your pregnancy, you'll probably be able to cut back your moisturizing routine—nature will take over and your skin's natural oils will (finally) give you that "special glow." (Start using the "Super Six" Base Prescription Sleep Serum for oily skin.)

But there's one possible skin complication of pregnancy you may not be aware of, chloasma, or the "mask of pregnancy," brown-pigmented blotches that appear on some women's faces (notably the dark- or olive-skinned) during pregnancy. These, like your waistline, will gradually diminish after your baby is born. In the meantime, should you get this splotched look, stay out of the sun—exposure to the ultraviolet rays will darken the patches even further. If you must go out in the sun, wear a strong sunblock. Cosmetic corrections for pigmentation problems are discussed in Part Six, Chapter 17.

PART FOUR

HOW TO RECYCLE AND REDESIGN YOUR BODY VIA DIET, EXERCISE, AND CAMOUFLAGE

CHAPTER 7

❦❦❦

The 24-Hour Emergency Diet: The Doctor's Healthful Way to Lose 2 to 5 Pounds in Just One Day

Have you ever had an *emergency call*, a jingle of the phone that resulted in your need to get thin super-fast? You know what I mean if a voice at the other end of the wire resulted in one of these I-feel-fat crises:

Emergency #1: Your ex-husband, whom you haven't seen since you handed him his toothbrush six months ago, wants to meet day after *tomorrow* to discuss the property settlement (and rumor has it he no longer has a corpulent midsection).

Emergency #2: Your ex-husband's new wife will be in town day after *tomorrow* to discuss the children's summer camp.

Emergency #3: A special man you haven't seen in ten years invites you to lunch day after *tomorrow*, and his visions of your body of yesteryear may be dashed over the apéritif if you can't drop a few pounds fast.

Emergency #4: The secretary of your college or high school graduating class just found your address, the reunion is day after *tomorrow*, won't you please come? (And you've been entertaining "if-they-could-see-me-now" fantasies for 15 years.)

You no longer have to turn down these last-minute invitations because I'm about to show you how New York beauties perform the seemingly impossible feat of losing 2 to 5 pounds in 24 hours. But first, now that I have your attention (if you aren't riveted to the page by the promise of instant weight loss, you're not a true diet fanatic!), I want to go over some weight-loss facts that will help you understand the instant-thin regimens so you can incorporate them into your own figure-reshaping plans.

If you're serious about recycling your body so you can project the image of a woman 10 years your junior, you probably think you really should a) diet, b) exercise, c) change the way you dress. If you picked one of the above, you're wrong. You can't choose *one:* You need a planned program combining *all three.* Especially if your carefully preserved senior prom corsage has long since crumbled to dust, it's no longer enough to jog 3 miles a day, curb your daily calories to 1,000, or encase yourself in a tent dress. Your body may demand more from you now, but if you know how to handle its changes, you don't have to be the less than proud owner of a shape that time is shifting floorward. (If you suddenly have become afflicted with terminal sag or a bit of free-floating flab, which has led to free-floating anxiety, you know what I mean.)

You're ready to reach for the hemlock but have decided to wait and share the potion with your entire bridge club? Poison is *not* the ℞ I had in mind. While I can't clone you with the firm flesh of an 18-year-old (beware beauty experts in pointed hats who guarantee magic cures!), I can show you how to fit yourself into a terrific 10-years-younger figure.

The first step to a recycled body is, as you might have guessed, diet. Unless you've been cloistered in a monastery since you left the cradle, I'm sure you've probably tried several "sure-fire" weight-loss programs already. And as you know, if you've spent any time in a bookstore lately, *the last thing America needs is another diet.* There are now more books dealing with weight loss than volumes detailing the rise and fall of the Roman Empire.

Yet at the beauty and success seminars I've hosted, the question of diet is sure to come up. And that question is most often asked by women who are no more than 5 to 15 pounds over their desired goal, sophisticated dieters who have tried everything from the most unsophisticated finger-down-the-throat plan to the great bran purge. That's why I say the last thing you need, if you've long since won your ribbons on the weight-loss battlefield, is another diet.

What you *really* need is a simple diet support system that works automatically and quickly with any diet that you find successful for your body and system. A support system that goes into high gear when the diet you've been following with success suddenly ceases working and your weight just won't budge. What causes a pounds-off program to grind to a halt this way? Or the most diligent dieters to grow so discouraged under such a circumstance that they "fall off the wagon"?

Diet Destroyer #1

Since all your sacrifice appears to be for nought, you start cheating. (If you've never had this experience, you've never been on a diet!)

Diet Destroyer #2

Since all your sacrifice appears to be for nought, you give up altogether!

Diet Destroyer #3

A psychological or emotional crisis strikes, and we go off our diets because we've:

- got a new lover (I'm so happy I could—and will—eat everything in sight)
- lost an old lover (I'm so miserable I could—and will—eat everything in sight)
- eaten American plan on vacation
- fed a cold too well when laid up in bed a few days
- celebrated the holidays with too much gusto
- attended a convention where business was conducted over breakfast-lunch-dinner
- etc., etc., etc.—you probably have your own favorite excuses

Even those women (and there were many) who reported success by following the healthful Sacred Cow Diet I outlined in my first book (wherein, briefly speaking, beef, booze, and salt were banned for 3 weeks and nutritious low-calorie substitutes were prescribed in their stead) felt the need for a change of routine now and then when their willpower—and weight loss—stalled in neutral.

What is the best way for a dieter to boost her spirits and start her weight going down once more? Forget a new dress and other temporary inducements. The best willpower booster I've found, one that will get you back on the wagon or help you get slim for a big occasion fast, is *the ability to lose 2 to 5 pounds in just one day, an ability you'll master by following the Instant 24-Hour Emergency! Diet.*

When I have a special occasion coming up, whether it's a TV appearance, an important meeting, or a special party, nothing makes me feel more ready for the big event than looking my best, which means looking my thinnest. But because I'm interested in healthful weight loss, I wouldn't attempt even a 24-hour diet without the advice of an expert.

For advice on the Instant 24-Hour Emergency! Diet, I went to Dr. Stanley Title, M.D., a well-known Manhattan weight-control specialist. You think you're the only one who worries about her body? Dr. Title's office is *filled* with 30-ish ballet dancers (yes, there are some, though you'd never guess it to look at them), models, stewardesses, and soap opera stars (these ladies of the afternoon don't try to look ingénue-young, but they certainly look glamorous)—women whose careers will fall by the wayside if their bodies fail to shape up. They seek help from Dr. Title and his associate, Dr. Charles Klein (a nutritionist with a Ph.D. from New York University), because these doctors emphasize a nutritional means to the good-looks end.

The following Emergency! diets are designed to be followed for one day at a time (they wouldn't be healthy over the long haul), but I think they're the perfect ℞ if you've reached a plateau, need to lose a few pounds fast, or if your weight is slowly returning even though you're still dieting. As Dr. Title explains, they are all also quite helpful in purifying and cleansing the system over the long haul—which means they get rid of the wastes that lead to less than clear, glowing (young) skin.

Note: When following any of the Instant 24-Hour Emergency! Diets, make sure you take your multivitamin and 1,000 mg vitamin C (500 mg in A.M., 500 in P.M.).

THE INSTANT PRE-LUNCH-WITH-YOUR-EX-HUSBAND 24-HOUR EMERGENCY! DIET

BREAKFAST

4 oz. tomato juice
Tea or coffee (may use 2 teaspoons skim milk)

MID-MORNING

2 glasses cold mineral water or sugar-free diet soda
Tea or coffee

LUNCH

⅓ cantaloupe melon *or* 1 medium tomato *or* 1 large cucumber *or* pickle
Diet soda

MID-AFTERNOON

Tall glass lemonade with sugar substitute (may repeat later in warm weather)

SUPPER

⅓ cantaloupe *or* 1 medium tomato *or* 1 large cucumber *or* pickle
4 oz. tomato juice
Tea or coffee

AFTER SUPPER

Diet gelatin or ⅓ cantaloupe

THE INSTANT PRE-LUNCH-WITH-YOUR-EX-HUSBAND'S-NEW-WIFE 24-HOUR EMERGENCY! DIET

BREAKFAST

½ grapefruit or ½ cantaloupe
Tea or coffee (black), 1 cup
     or
4 oz. orange juice or ½ grapefruit or ½ cantaloupe
1 cup cooked brown rice (no salt)
Medium orange
Tea or coffee (black), 1 cup

LUNCH

1 cup cooked brown rice (no salt)
⅓ grapefruit
½ cup water-packed canned fruit or fresh fruit

SUPPER

1 cup cooked brown rice (no salt)
4 oz. prune juice or orange juice
½ cantaloupe or 1 medium apple or pear
Tea or coffee (black)

℞ *for cheaters*. You may top rice with 1 teaspoon honey or soy sauce.

THE INSTANT I-HAVEN'T-SEEN-HIM-IN-10-YEARS 24-HOUR EMERGENCY! DIET

The following 2-to-5-pound instant weight-loss plans will appeal to those of you who prefer to eat whenever you're hungry, rather than waiting for prescribed meal and snack times. When you practice the following fruit/vegetable alternatives, you are also allowed all the coffees, teas, diet and club sodas, and water you desire (but no juices).

The 24-Hour Apple Fruit Boost

Up to 6 medium apples a day (if you're hungriest in the morning, for example, have 2 for breakfast, 1 each in the mid-morning, at lunchtime, in the mid-afternoon, and for supper. If lunch is your *fall off the wagon* time, have 2 at noon.) Eat them either raw or baked (the latter are easier to digest).

You are also allowed unlimited coffees, teas, diet and club sodas, and water (but no juices).

℞ *for cheaters.* If your hunger becomes uncontrollable, add a third of a head of lettuce to your apples-and-liquid regimen.

℞ *for "cheater" cheaters.* Remember how he used to call you "the body beautiful" 10 years ago? Think before you add even a lettuce leaf to your intake!

Apple Alternatives

You can substitute the following fruits for apples, dividing the intake throughout the day, according to your appetite:
up to 3 medium cantaloupes
   or
up to 6 medium bananas
   or
up to 6 medium grapefruits
   or
up to 10 cups strawberries (be careful; some people are very allergic to strawberries)
   or
up to 8 oranges

The Semi-Vegetable Alternative

Combine half the amount of any of the above fruits, plus all the sugar-free liquids listed on page 100 (except juice), with up to a head of lettuce and up to 3 stalks of celery for the day.

THE INSTANT PRE-REUNION 24-HOUR EMERGENCY! DIET

BREAKFAST

4 oz. grapefruit juice or orange juice (unsweetened)
Tea or coffee (may use 2 teaspoons skim milk)

MID-MORNING

2 glasses cold mineral water or sugar-free diet soda
Tea or coffee

LUNCH

Hot clear chicken soup or beef broth
Diet soda (sugar free)

MID-AFTERNOON

Tall glass lemonade with sugar substitute (may repeat later in warm
  weather)

SUPPER

Diet gelatin
4 oz. grapefruit juice (unsweetened)
Tea or coffee

AFTER SUPPER

Diet soda
Diet gelatin
4 oz. grapefruit or orange juice (or 1 cup beef or chicken bouillon)

℞ *for cheaters.* If your cravings for solid food become unbearable later on in the day or evening, you can "cheat" with any combination of lettuce, cucumbers, radishes, and/or celery (not to exceed more than 2 medium-size salad bowls a day) dressed with lemon juice, vinegar, or 1 teaspoon diet dressing.

No doubt about it, the above Instant 24-Hour Emergency! Diets involve sacrifice, but the beauty is that the sacrifice is only for a short period, and the pounds you can lose might take far longer on an ordinary diet. Still, if you find your hands trembling and your throat turning dry at the thought of limiting your food intake, start by going on the Emergency! diet for *half a day*, gradually building up to a full day. And remember, these are special-occasion diets to *help you give a nudge to your own weight-loss program*. Don't follow them more often than once a week unless you are under a doctor's care.

But to show you that diet doctors do have a heart (lean and strong, no doubt) and they do understand a craving for sweets, you can add the delicious recipe below to any of the instant diets without throwing your 24-hour weight loss out of whack.

Dr. Title's Emergency! Diet Frappé

Pour ¼ cup 99-percent-fat-free milk into an 8-ounce glass. Cover with chilled, just opened (freshly carbonated) diet soda: No-Cal chocolate, No-Cal cream (for a vanilla flavor), or Cott's chocolate cherry diet soda. The drink will foam up like a calorie-laden soda fountain concoction. The carbonation will give you a full feeling, and the flavorings will satisfy your sweet tooth. Drink in the evening, after supper.

THIN ISN'T ENOUGH

When the Duchess of Windsor said, "You can't be too rich or too thin," she should have added, "but you can be too wrinkled." Especially if you're over 30. There is another part to the post-puberty diet story that hasn't been told before. That is: Thin is not enough. Too many dieted, trim bodies are topped by faces that are dehydrated, consequently haggard looking. You need a firm, sleek body that's topped by a smooth, unlined face, and to get both you need a long-term diet aid that will help you counteract the haggard look that a diet can induce.

This long-term diet aid is readily available. What is it? Simply . . . water, a magical elixir that can help you shed pounds while you plump up your skin. And in some specific instances, mineral water. I will explain.

The Well-Watered Body: Some Like It Hard

The following 9-word statement is really a can't-fail stay-thin Rx that will help you become 10 pounds thinner and look 10 years younger.

Drink six 8-ounce glasses of water every day. Follow this advice, and the price you've paid for this book will pay for itself in body-saving dividends. Why? Water will fill you up, curb your appetite, and hydrate your cells while adding zero calories to your waistline.

I work with thin models every day and see them at professional parties, and whether they're holding a Styrofoam cup or a Waterford goblet, I assure you these young-looking beauties are not guzzling foaming pink alcohol-laden concoctions topped with little paper parasols. They *are* sipping water. Constantly. The first secret every newcomer is taught when she signs on with a model agency is, "*Do* go near the water." Not only are these well-watered women cutting calories, they are also cleansing their systems via a good flow of H_2O.

What *kind* of water should you swallow? Believe it or not, water is *not* just water. And yes, I do believe you are what you drink—the state of your health (not to mention your shape) can be influenced by the water you sip. You should be drinking *hard*, not soft, water. (The latter makes washing your hair and dishes easier, but it's not as helpful to drink as hard water.) Hard water means mineral-rich water, heavy in calcium and magnesium, among other important elements. A diet rich in hard water will keep you feeling, as well as looking, young, because it helps prevent hardening of the arteries, high blood pressure, heart disease—a whole range of cardiovascular problems. Some gerontologists believe that in the Hunza valley of the Himalayas, where centenarians are almost as common as diet experts are here, the people's reliance on highly mineralized water is closely linked to their long, productive life spans.

How do you know exactly what you're drinking? Call your local water department for a *grain* analysis. No, there is no wheat coming out of the tap (at least we hope not!). You want the number of grains of calcium and magnesium per gallon of H_2O (0–3 grains per gallon = soft water; 4–10 grains per gallon = hard; 11–19 grains = very hard).

If the water is hard but you don't like the taste, baby yourself. Pediatricians urge mothers of newborns to boil (sterilize) the infants' drinking water before serving. Boil your own drinking supply for 5 minutes, let cool, and the taste (not to mention the quality) should improve.

Your water department says you would have to submerge yourself in the local reservoir for days to up your mineral intake? You're a candidate for bottled mineral water. (Note: I said mineral, not distilled water. The latter may be ultra-pure, but in the process of making it so, they've taken out the minerals, which makes drinking distilled water ultra-ridiculous—not to mention tasteless. Save distilled water for machines that call for it—your steam iron, for example. We use distilled water in our salon facial apparatus—it's sediment- and mineral-free, so it won't gum up the works.) Bottled mineral waters are not free, but since you're not indulging in expensive diet gimmickry (from rainbow-colored pills that speed up your ill humor instead of your weight loss, to Texas grapefruit flown up out of season by Lear jet), you deserve to make your water cure something you'll enjoy.

Here is what my mineral water maintenance involves: I want you to drink at least six 8-ounce glasses (more whenever you're thirsty) a day, at the following times: one when you awake in the morning, one before lunch, one at 3 P.M. (or whenever your mid-afternoon hunger pangs strike), two glasses before dinner, one before bed. Naturally, the amount of mineral water you substitute for tap H$_2$O will be pegged to your budget, but do try for at least three helpings of the bottled variety daily.

Now, I'm not talking about replacing *all* your food with water (that's total fasting, which could fast become boring, as well as make you both weak-kneed and weak-headed). Just drink your mineral water before the meals prescribed by your own diet plan, and you will be more successful at your weight-loss attempts. It sounds simple, but it will work, especially if you indulge in a little psychological game-playing. To keep up your water regimen, you have to convince yourself that what you're drinking is a treat, not a chore. That is one reason why I recommend mineral waters; they taste better than the tap variety, and if you vary the brands you try, you may find yourself looking forward to an import like Perrier before lunch, or Saratoga, a bubbly domestic, for dinner (though I doubt if even the ultra-chic sit around saying, ". . . a delightful little mineral water with a lovely hint of limestone; it must come from the northern side of the rock fissure").

Here, some prescriptions for making mineral water part of your permanent slash-10-years program:

℞. *Don't cheat yourself.* True, just about everything (including our bodies) contains water. An apple is 85 percent H$_2$O; bread is 33 percent water. Coffee, tea, and soft drinks are liquid, too. But when I talk about six glasses a day, I'm talking about straight water—not coffee or tea (and you *cannot* wring out your toast!) for those times when your water is scheduled. If you want to watch those pounds disappear and a smooth, young-looking face appear, you have to be serious about your water.

℞. *If you're suffering from unbounded girth but have yet to develop unbounded thirst,* you may well be wondering, "Is there nothing I can mix with water that will count toward my six a day?" You *can* mix your chosen water with natural fruit juice, a wonderful taste additive. Pair your morning nonbubbly water with a few tablespoons of orange, grapefruit, pineapple juice—whatever will help you get the water down before meals.

℞. *When you ban the booze, substitute the bubbly.* Since alcohol is fattening (not to mention aging to skin and body) and water is the opposite, serve yourself a sparkling mineral water once or twice a day instead of a drink. Sweeten your sparkling water with a few tablespoons of grape juice and you will feel as though you're drinking a wine spritzer, a popular summer drink. Or take it straight with a twist of lemon or lime, and your sparkling water will be a true *à votre santé* cocktail.

Mineral Water Shopping List

Sophisticated Europeans eliminated tap water from their diet years ago. The American thirst for mineralized H_2O is in its infancy by comparison. If you're wondering which varieties to sample, you might want to begin with what is probably the world's best selling, Evian. This still water is practically sodium (salt) free, and it's got a refreshing, clear taste. Vichy Célestine (bubbly), Vittel (still), and Perrier (very bubbly) are other popular French imports.

Fiuggi (still) is the best-known Italian water. San Peliegrino (bubbles added) is a close second.

On the home front, Mountain Valley (still) has been quaffed since De Soto toured what is now Hot Springs, Arkansas, back in 1541. Saratoga and Poland Spring are two additional native American waters you might want to try. But don't limit yourself. Different parts of the country have excellent regional waters well worth testing.

Water: the Ultimate Skin Booster

I've just discussed how a water regimen will help you drop pounds by curbing your appetite. Now, how will H_2O take years from your face?

In the previous chapters I mentioned the importance of hydrating your skin externally—feeding it water from the outside. (Remember, young-looking skin equals moist-looking skin—and you can have it at any age.) But you must also water your skin *internally*, and that's where mineral water maintenance plays a significant role. Because while you're unclogging your arteries, detoxifying your system (water helps wash out dirt and poisons), and de-escalating your appetite, the water you're drinking will also be filling up your cells from the inside and giving your face a fresh, moist, smooth look. If you diet "dry" (without taking enough water), your skin will look wrinkled and baggy because it will have nothing soft and springy to rest on. As Dr. Klein explains, the crepey-skinned look that many dieters experience is not due solely to loss of muscle tone—it's also caused by dehydration. Most of us have known dieters who really looked better fat. No matter how sleek you've made your body, if it must coexist with a dehydrated, drawn face, you'll look older than you should, not younger. (You don't look a day over 37? Terrific, unless you're 27!)

INFORMATION PLEASE

Before I leave the subject of both short-term and lifetime weight loss, I want to answer specific diet questions I'm often asked.

🌀 *Re: Mineral water maintenance. Should I drink bubbly or still?*

Carbon dioxide gas makes mineral waters bubbly—but it can also give you that bloated, gassy feeling if you drink too much. I drink one glass of the bubbly variety (which I think has more flavor and is more fun) before lunch, a second as part of my two glasses before dinner, unless it's a day I'm following my 24-Hour Emergency! Diet, in which case I forgo my predinner mineral water for Dr. Title's postprandial Emergency! Diet Frappé.

🌀 *I'm eating the same amount I did 10 years ago and exercising just as much, yet I'm gaining weight. How come?*

Though you *think* you haven't slowed down since you were 18, your metabolism has, which means your body is no longer processing the nutrients and calories you take in with all deliberate speed. An adult male (sometimes I think those two words are a contradiction) who weighs in at 150 when he's 30 years old will tip the scale at 200 when he's 60 if he doesn't cut back from his 30-year-old calorie intake. The older we get, the less we should consume to maintain our ideal weight. So if you're ingesting the same number of calories you did 10 years ago, you're not keeping pace with the inevitable internal bodily slowdown. The only solution is to reduce the quantity of food you eat.

While I'm not a member of the sugar lobby, I do have a sweet tooth. What harm will a teaspoon or two a day do? I'm no longer at the cavity-prone stage.

Sounds like your store of nutritional knowledge is not as ample as your caloric intake; you probaby had the same sparse junior high home economics food training as I did. Hopefully, nutrition education has advanced since then, but here are a few postgraduate sugar nuggets to digest before you lift your next teaspoon:

The average American consumes some *18,000 pounds of sugar* in his/her lifetime.

Even if you cut out your sugar in coffee, you may not be aware of the enormous amounts of the sweetener you are still consuming. *Consumer Reports* tells us that Jell-O contains 82.6 percent sugar; Quaker Natural Cereal is 23.9 percent sugar; Shake 'n Bake Barbecue Chicken coating is 50.9 percent sugar. Understand that the label may not say "sugar"—but if the product includes sucrose, corn sugar, corn syrup, maltose, or dextrose, it's all sugar by another name.

The reason the above is bad (besides the fact that sugar contains non-productive, empty calories) is that your sugar tooth robs the body of B vitamins (crucial for blood and beauty) in two ways. As Dr. Klein explains, it prevents absorption of the B factors and triggers insulin production, which is also harmful to Bs.

I've always envied those skinny models in fashion magazines, so I've thinned myself down to a size 8. I'm tall and attractive—why do I look more ghoulish than gorgeous?

How old are you? Those sexy-yet-string-bean-thin models are usually 18 to 23 years old. You see, when you're that young (and have been that thin most of your life), you don't need any padding on your form or on your face, because there are no wrinkles or sags that need filling up. That's why modeling is a young woman's business. By the time these elegant creatures turn 30, they have three options: 1) gain a little weight and start hawking housewifely products like floor wax; 2) live off what they've saved of the six-figure incomes they've been earning since their late teens; 3) marry a fabulously wealthy doctor or real estate entrepreneur. Clever they are, so most of them seem to opt for number 3 (can you blame them?). Of course, there are exceptions—superstar models who stay on top until (by modeling standards) their dotage, that is, 34 years old. But as a top photographer told me, you can be sure it takes longer to photograph these famous faces (special lighting and specially angled poses are needed) than it did when these same women were fresh-faced, wrinkle-free 21-year-olds.

But for the rest of us, the terribly thin look is not a desirable goal. Emaciation is aging. If you're over 35, a few extra pounds will keep you from looking brittle, keep your face from looking drained, and keep your breasts from emptying out.

After what seems like a lifetime of trying, I have finally reached my ideal weight, but those insurance company charts don't tell what to do if you're still out of proportion—my hips and thighs look as chunky today as they did when I wore a ruffled-panty size 3x sunsuit.

If only our brain could trigger our metabolism to lose the pounds where they need to be lost. Unfortunately, dieting is not a simple matter. The sad (if you're a sedentary sort like me) truth is *diet alone won't solve all figure problems*. You must exercise—diligently—those areas that need trimming and firming. And even exercise might not do it all.

If heavyset hips, et cetera, are noticeable way back at the beginning of your family album, *total* reproportioning may not be possible. Blame your disproportion on heredity, then start exercising to minimize the problem, which can be done. (It could be worse! Consider being stuck with the rumored Hapsburg *tail*, a much more bizarre familial trait than an ample bottom.)

The chapters that follow will tell you how to recycle your still less than perfect (welcome to the real world with the rest of us!) figure through a carefully designed body-lifting and camouflaging program.

CHAPTER 8

❦❦❦

The 10-Minute-a-Day 10-Years-Off
Tuneup That Reshapes You
through Body-Lifting (and Camouflage)

Your body, no matter what your mirror tells you, is a marvelous machine. It's got a terrific pump (your heart) that works nonstop; it runs efficiently when fed the right fuel (food/vitamins) and sufficient high-quality water. But even if you keep your motor in gear via perpetual motion endeavors like jumping rope or jogging (more about these later), your body may be beginning to resemble a clunky Edsel rather than a sleek Jaguar!

Once you reach the age of 25, your figure starts to change, starts to show signs of that dirty five-letter word, a-g-i-n-g. (Consolation: At least we don't rust!) At first the signs are subtle and you may not be aware of what is happening. You will notice: a) your clothes no longer fit quite right even though you still wear the same size; b) the appearance of a few dents, dimples, and bulges on your fenders that make you look as though you've been around the track once too often. You're ready to swallow a can of motor oil? Leave the STP to Le Mans competitors and learn how to re-engineer/redesign your shape via some clever Body-Lifting work.

To retool your chassis, you have to attack the trouble areas, those nasty body sags that proclaim you've put a few miles on your own personal speedometer. Remember, you can be underweight and under 30 and still have less than firm flesh. Nothing ages a woman faster.

What happens if you continue to chug merrily along, convinced that *your* body never will show these changes? Take the following True/False quiz for a preview of the future shlock that could occur if you don't adopt a regimen such as the simple anti-aging Body-Lifting program I will outline.

On a separate sheet of paper write the numbers of the questions below and mark True or False after each, then check your score against the paragraph that follows.

Future "Shlock" Body Quiz

1. When I raise my hand, my upper arm kind of hangs there—twisting slowly, slowly in the wind—and there's no breeze. True or False

2. The Last Time I Saw Paris was as a backpacking, hitchhiking student circa 1968. The last time I noticed my waist was that same summer, when I started a lifelong love affair with croissants and French bread. True or False

3. From the front, I'm in good shape. A side view might convince a just-earned-his-shingle obstetrician I'm three months pregnant, though I'm not. My 30th birthday has brought with it a pot belly. True or False

4. I'm considering taking up horse-riding—might as well put those saddlebag bulges draped over my outer thighs to good use. True or False

5. Rather than my legs swinging sexily when I walk, my inner thighs jiggle, making my nerves jangle. True or False

6. In the process of losing weight, I seem to have misplaced my breasts! They used to be small and firm, now they're empty and low, and I'm too old for a training bra. True or False

If you've answered more than one of the above questions True, you have at least one body flaw that may be aging you prematurely. Check the Body-Lift plan that follows and dwell on the routine geared to counteract your problem. If you're ambitious, do the others as well and you may prevent further figure flaws from doing damage (psychological as well as physical) to your shape. Remember, you'll be moving muscles that don't usually get a workout, so give yourself 6 weeks to see results.

What happens if your Body-Lifting doesn't bring about total improvement? If you're suffering from *plus ça change, plus c'est la même chose* (to rephrase the French, the more you change your exercise habits, the more you see the same body), then you have to take another tack.

I'll show you how to hide when you have tried, tried, tried . . . and your body flaw stubbornly refuses to disappear.

Because I'm a realist who knows from experience that a physical workout alone won't change everything, I know that after you work to correct body flaws via diet and exercise, you must use your head in the form of clever camouflage tricks to accomplish the rest. That is why I will treat every body problem with *two* solutions. First, Body-Lifting; second, Camouflage. The camouflage ideas will help you project an image of firm, well-proportioned flesh.

THE TODAY WOMAN'S WAY TO BRING BACK YESTERDAY'S BODY

Even before you cross the Great Divide into your 30s, your body is starting slowly to surrender to the forces of gravity. That's why slimming is no longer enough. Your new goal is firming, tightening, and *lifting* every part of your anatomy.

The face-lift has long since come out of the closet. Now, it's the era of the *Body-Lift*—a new standard in beauty-keeping body-rejuvenating fitness.

You say it sounds great but you're less than enthusiastic at the prospect of moving dormant muscles?

When it comes to exercise, I'll assume you're like me. Your flesh is *not* willing, and your willpower is weak. In other words, you're thinking of skipping this section, and you're guiltily promising yourself you'll diligently study the next chapter, even if it's a detailed discourse on the songs and mating rituals of the humpback whale (it isn't).

But you complain that even when you *do* exercise, it doesn't work? Probably (using my own anti-exercise bias as a guide) because you only *think* you're working out. If you slowly lift your arms as if to swat flies and manage barely to get your legs off the floor when your instructor's toes are reaching for the stars, you're practicing an exercise in self-delusion.

To make your body-work effective you have to expend *real effort*. So in order to make sure you don't cheat yourself and do get maximum lifting and firming in a minimum of time, I'm going to ask you to make a smart investment in a set of 3-pound dumbbells and 2-pound ankle weights (you'll find both at any sporting goods store for under fifteen dollars).

By lifting weights while you move, you'll be *forcing yourself* to get something out of your exercise session. (Obviously, if your arm is in the air and your weight is still on the floor, you can't convince yourself you're trying.)

You're worried that weight lifting will turn you into a contender for Olympic gold? Don't be. You're not going to learn to press 500-pound barbells—we'll leave that to the experts. You will use the light weights effectively to turn flab into firm flesh, then lift your newly firm flesh back where it was meant to be. By following the simple weight-training, shape-gaining exercises I prescribe, you actually will be toning and repositioning the fleshier parts of your body.

Before the instructions, here are a few quick exercise Q's and A's.

❧ *You say weight lifting will turn flab into "firm flesh" . . . doesn't that mean muscle?*

Yes, it means a little bit of muscle—that's what makes you look firm. The anemic, looks-like-she-can't-lift-a-fork look is out. What is in: a look of vitality (and, yes, strength). But these weights are so light by power-lifting standards there is no way you will turn into Arnold Schwarzenegger's long-lost twin. If you're still worried, understand that women don't produce enough of the male hormone testosterone to develop the bulk associated with pumping iron. One more plus for firm flesh: *Muscle takes less physical space than fat, so the trimmer you get, the more you lose in inches.*

❧ *I've never been fat and flabby. But as I've gotten older, what flesh I do have is starting to hang because I'm loose and too skinny. Doesn't that mean I'll exercise into nothingness with weights?*

You won't become The Incredible Shrinking Woman, but your lack of routinized exercise has already led to Incredible Shrinking Muscles. In your case, mini weight training won't be trading muscle for flab, it will be building firmer flesh where *nothing* now exists, so you will be developing a stronger, more filled-out look.

❧ *Are Body-Lifting exercises all I will need to recycle my figure into a 10-years-younger, 10-times-firmer form?*

No.

Sorry about that!

Since good health equals beauty, and a healthy heart and lungs equal good health, your beauty ℞ equation must include some form of aerobic exercise.

Rope skipping is my personal favorite, because you can do it anyplace and it takes a minimal investment of money and of time—*5 days a week, 5 minutes a day, 500 skips nonstop* will benefit your entire cardiovascular system (not to mention your legs). But build to that 500 goal very slowly—jumping rope is a strenuous exercise, especially if you're out of shape. Start with no more than 25 skips per session. I'm especially fond of jumping rope because it attacks my own personal nemesis: 5 extra pounds clinging to my hips.

You don't need me to tell you the benefits of jogging. You probably have more than one friend more than willing to sing the praises of this discipline. As far as making you look 10 years younger, jogging will help build up endurance, strength, and physical fitness, so you will feel good. And if you feel good, you really do look good (pardon my cliché)—that's what exercising to look younger is all about.

But if you're 30-plus and the gulf between your stay-put life and running seems like a veritable chasm, you can bridge the gap with an exercise discipline that even the laziest can learn to love: *walking*.

That's right, this most mundane of activities, when practiced correctly (that is, aerobically), can boost your fitness level (not to mention increase your heart and lung efficiency). But you can't just stroll along smelling the flowers! You have to expend some real effort to get real results. *Walk briskly*, spine erect, arms swinging in a natural rhythm. Wear running shoes to cushion your feet.

Fifteen minutes of nonstop brisk walking a day (build up to it slowly, especially if you're out of shape) will help you build strength *and* vitality. You increase your speed as your endurance builds up. When you find your current brisk pace no more invigorating than a nonaerobic saunter, start walking to a faster rhythm. You're walking too fast if: 1) you're breathless, 2) you're painfully uncomfortable, 3) you can't carry on a normal conversation with a companion. (You're alone? If you can't recite your favorite poem —or your marketing list—without sounding like an ailing frog, you know it's time to slow down.)

Many former joggers (running can lead to foot and leg injuries if you're not careful) are becoming fitness walkers. In fact, I wouldn't be surprised if the jogging paths are soon filled with walkers giving the runners a run for their money!

Just remember to check with your doctor before you begin aerobic exercises, or the Body-Lift program that follows.

I understand the relationship between dieting *and calories; what about exercise and caloric intake?*

Every food is granted a certain caloric count. As you know, it takes 3,500 calories to equal a pound—therefore, to lose one pound you cut 3,500 calories from your diet. Of course, you can't cut out calories completely— starvation can be hazardous to your health. What you must do is burn up the excess calories that would ordinarily be stored in your body as fat. Self-immolation is not the perfect method of calorie burning—you have to exercise. A physical workout creates the energy that burns away the excess calories that turn into fat. As you inch up the age scale and your metabolism slows down, you must also push up your energy outflow. More exercise (as well as fewer calories) will compensate for a slowing metabolism.

THE BODY-LIFT VIA WEIGHT TRAINING AND CLOTHES CAMOUFLAGE WORKSHOP

℞ FOR BEGINNERS:

Warm up. Don't expect your "engine" to go from zero to full throttle without letting it rev up first. Five minutes' worth of stretching activities will do (try arm swings, shaking out both your legs, bending from the waist with bouncing motions to reach for your toes, 60 seconds of in-place jogging). To cool down when you're finished, do more stretching and walk around for a few minutes before heading for the nearest chair.

Fit Body-Lifting into your daily routine (the exercises won't take long and they will be easier to remember if they become a habit).

The first three days you perform the lifts, do them without weights so your body will become accustomed to the workout before it becomes a bit more strenuous.

Back problems? Don't do any exercises without checking with your M.D. or physical therapist.

℞ TO FIRM AND LIFT FLESHY UPPER ARMS:

Holding a weight in each hand, place feet comfortably together, stand erect, and raise your arms straight ahead to shoulder level (see illustration, position 1). Swing arms up to the ceiling and return to straight-ahead position. Repeat 10 times; return to starting position. Now, swing arms back behind you as close to straight back as you can get (position 2). Repeat 10 times in this position.

This exercise also helps strengthen the muscles of the chest wall (important to give the illusion of a firmer bustline) and helps improve the contour of *scrawny* upper arms as well. Remember, thin isn't everything—shape is the key.

℞ TO CAMOUFLAGE LESS THAN FIRM UPPER ARMS:

The last time I had a variety of sleeveless tops in my closet? About the same time I looked forward to after-school milk and cookies.

Avoid sleeveless and tank tops, halters and strapless tube tops.

Short sleeves look less than terrific on most women; they emphasize arm thickness, thinness, or looseness. Exception: A short, nonfitting sleeve that

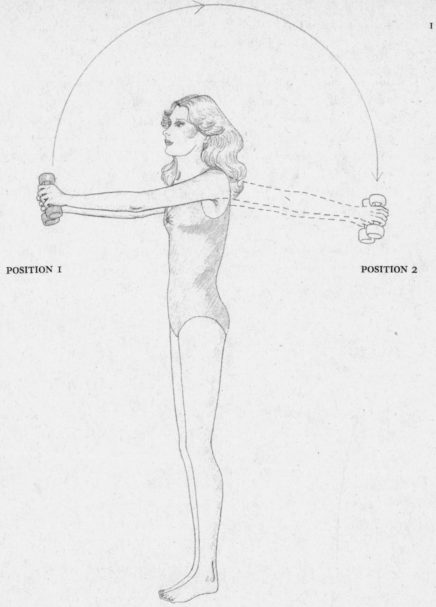

POSITION I   POSITION 2

reaches almost to your elbow (the kind of short, fluttery sleeve found on sheer summer dresses).

Cheat your way to a short-sleeved look by rolling long sleeves up to a point just below your elbow. (While you're at it, have you looked at your elbows lately? They do wrinkle. Make it a point to cream them with body lotion/oil during and after your bath.)

Draw attention away from your upper arm with interesting bracelets on your wrist.

Long sleeves are best. But tight and long will make your arm look like a stuffed sausage. A soft, flowing sleeve that tapers and buttons at the wrist is a good bet.

℞ TO FIRM THE BOSOM:

Because exercise firms muscles and the bosom itself is made of fatty tissue, exercise won't firm the bosom *per se*. It *will* strengthen the pectoral muscles, which underlie and support the breasts, which in turn can give you a slightly firmer look. When it comes to changing breast shape, camouflage and under-wear are better solutions. So is good posture: Check your breasts in a side-view mirror a) while you slouch, b) standing up straight. Your whole body will look 10 years younger and pounds thinner if you stand correctly. If you want to do what you can to correct sag via Body-Lifting, try this one for your "pecs."

Lie on floor, swing arms straight up, dumbbell in each hand (position 1). Bring weights toward chest, hold above chest for count of 1 (position 2), raise arms to ceiling again, hold for count of 1. Repeat 10 times.

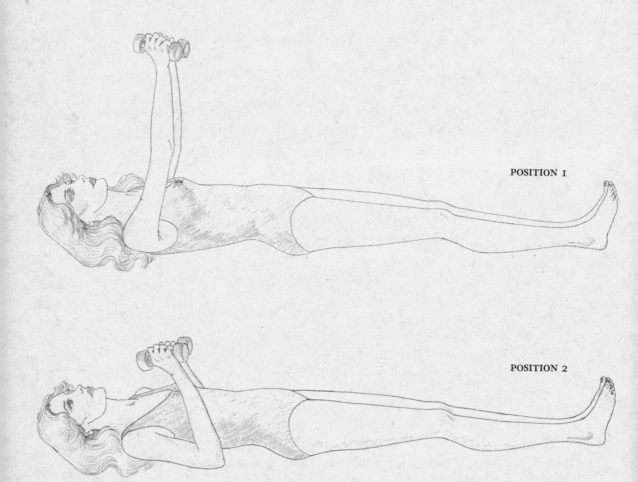

POSITION 1

POSITION 2

℞ TO CAMOUFLAGE AND MINIMIZE THE BOSOM THAT'S TOO LARGE (START-ING TO LOOK MATRONLY):

When you're young, full breasts are certainly no problem and can actually enhance (though for dubious reasons) the popularity of the high school girl. But as you get older, large can look matronly if you're not care-ful, and a large, sagging bosom looks worse than the smaller variety. Besides, bosom styles change, and the sexy, overpowering Mae West big bosom is not today's ideal. If your bosom is starting to become a little pendulous, do the following:

Avoid clinging tops. It's obvious to everyone that you've got it. You don't have to flaunt it. A loosely fitting silk shirt will project your message tastefully.

Make sure jewelry doesn't hang over the edge of your bosom. Wear medium-sized pieces rather than teeny-tiny pins or huge, overpowering necklaces.

Beware the wide, stiff belt. It will make you look as if you have no midriff at all.

Stay away from double-breasted jackets. Even if you're just 25, these will make you look stodgy and thick-waisted.

You don't have to give up sweaters; just make sure the style you choose has a little "give." The skin-tight sweater (the look that wowed them 20 years ago), no matter how soft and elegant the fabric, is no longer for you.

The right bra is your years-younger godsend. See the following chapter.

℞ TO CAMOUFLAGE AND ENHANCE A SMALL BOSOM THAT'S LOST ITS SHAPE AS YOU'VE GOTTEN OLDER (DUE TO CONSTANT DIETING, BABIES, GRAVITY):

Wear shirts with lots of detail: yokes, shirring, pockets; flowing peasant-style blouses; patterned tops.

While you can wear flowing-type shirts, don't wear something so large that it's baggy—you'll look totally shapeless.

Softly fitting sweaters will look good—just avoid the tightest of clings, as well as vertically narrow-ribbed styles.

Double-breasted jackets will give you added dimension up top.

Wear the right bra and too small really will be no problem at all. (See next chapter.)

℞ TO TRIM WAIST AND MIDRIFF:

Stand with legs about 12 inches apart, knees slightly bent, arms holding weights at your sides. Slowly bend sideways (not forward) at the waist, letting your right hand inch down your right leg, your left arm and hand rise and curve over your head. Keeping your feet on the floor, bounce your

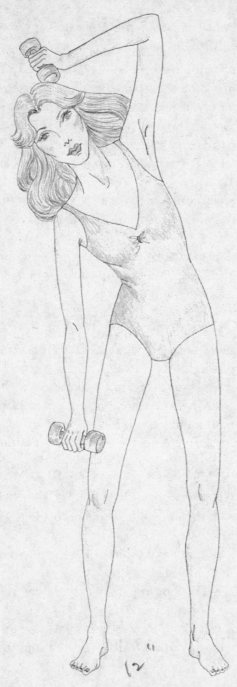

body 3 times to the right. Reverse arm placement and bounce 3 times to the left. As you inch arm lower down each leg, feel the other side of your waist/torso stretch. Repeat series 10 times each side, making sure your knees stay bent and your body doesn't tip forward.

℞ TO CAMOUFLAGE LARGE WAIST AND MIDRIFF:

Don't draw attention to your waist by wearing clothes that contrast in the middle, such as black pants and a white top. Instead, pick shades of one color in a two-piece outfit. If there is a definite contrast between two pieces you *love* and so must wear, turn a tucked-in shirt into a blouson—if it curves softly over the waist, your waist won't be quite so obvious.

Long sweaters and tunics look terrific, hide waistline and bulging midriff with flair.

Don't follow fashion if it dictates wide cummerbund-type belts, belts made of shiny fabric, or cinchers festooned with glittering stones.

Choose narrow, strippy belts or buckle belts about one inch wide.

A narrow, dark leather belt tied over a slightly blousy silk shirt that's worn over your skirt or slacks offers good camouflage.

Clingy jersey or knit dresses that hug your midriff and pinch at your waist are out.

Exception: A clingy jersey is in if you layer said dress with a sleeveless tunic or vest to get the long, sexy look and feel of a soft fabric without its body-revealing drawbacks.

Choose skirts and trousers with a narrow (or nonexistent) waistband.

Get rid of belt loops. They add inches to your waist.

Check the underwear chapter that follows.

℞ TO FLATTEN A SAGGING TUMMY:

Lie on your back on the floor, legs resting on floor in front of you, arms at your sides, palms down. Lift your legs, holding them straight, no more than 3 inches off the floor; hold for 30 seconds. Lower. (It may take you awhile to maintain the position for 30 seconds.) Repeat 3 times. You will feel a tightening of the inner thighs as well as of the abdomen when you do this exercise.

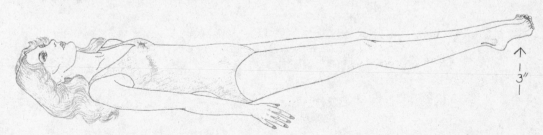

Since I hear "How can I get a flat stomach?" so often (stomach muscles are worked so little they can weaken, loosen, and fall), I'll add one more exercise for the ambitious.

℞ TO LIFT AND FLATTEN A SAGGING TUMMY, PART II

Stand with feet planted well apart, so you feel you're balanced on a firm foundation. Holding weights, lift arms up and out at your sides, so hands are level with shoulders. Without moving your feet and legs, slowly twist torso as far to the left as possible. Your left hand will naturally swing behind you, your right arm should swing in front of you. Now, twist torso to the right; your right arm swings behind you, your left arm in front of you. Keep legs in same position, repeat exercise 10 times, alternating sides. The repetitions should form one continuous, rhythmic movement.

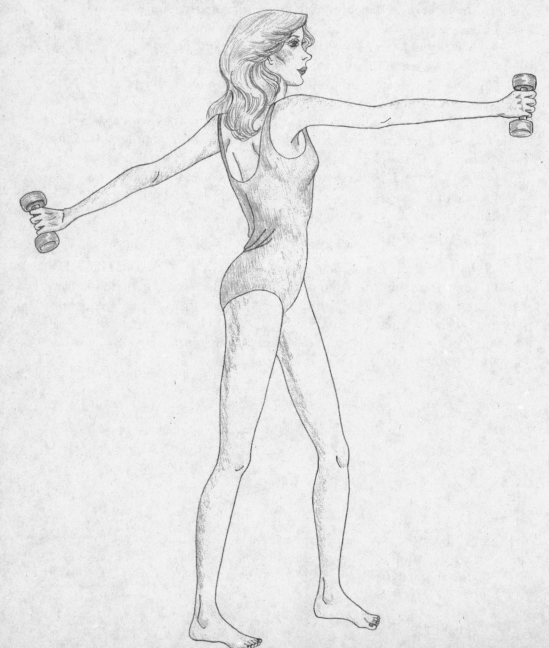

℞ TO CAMOUFLAGE A PROTRUDING STOMACH:

Avoid gathered, dirndl-type skirts. They don't conceal, they accentuate.
Look for skirts with darts or stitching over the stomach. Skirts that are stitched down over the stomach hang more smoothly.

Straight skirts and clingy fabrics won't look good from the side. Variations of the A-line are still your best friend; a slightly flared (not voluminous) skirt or dress will be a close second.

The long sweater or tunic will hide, after you've tried, tried, tried, and the bulge just won't go away.

Donate any skirt or pants with embroidery, front zipper, or front pockets to the Salvation Army.

Don't tuck in sweaters or shirts if the fabric bunches up over your stomach.

Check the next chapter for everything you must know about undergarments.

℞ TO DEBULGE OUTER THIGHS:

Wearing ankle weights, lie on side as illustrated with legs straight at an angle slightly in front of your hips. Raise top leg as high as you can (it won't be very high at first), keeping outer thigh toward ceiling, knee and toe pointing forward. Lift your bottom leg till it joins top leg. Hold for count of 3. Slowly lower bottom leg; lower top leg till you're back at the starting position. Repeat 10 times on each side of the body.

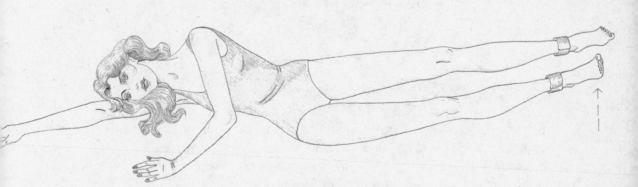

℞ TO SLIM OUTER THIGHS (AND MAKE HIPS LOOK NARROWER) VIA CAMOUFLAGE:

Trick the eye by drawing attention away from your bottom half. A blouson top will make you look better proportioned; so will necklaces, scarves tied at the throat or over the bust, an interesting neckline.

A-line skirts work, and if your stomach is small, a gathered dirndl will move the eye away from your outer silhouette toward the center.

You can wear pants, but clingy polyester is out: It accentuates every oversized curve. And don't think you're camouflaging by wearing a matching polyester jacket. The solid polyester pantsuit is definitely matronly; it also signifies lack of flair.

Instead of the polyester pantsuit, top a pair of well-cut natural fiber (wool, cotton blend, gabardine) pants that hang straight and loose from the buttocks (check yourself in a side-view mirror: if the pants "cup" your derrière, they're not for you) with a blouson, or layer on a young-looking accessory like a vest.

The dress rule mimics the skirt caveat: A straight, clingy style that outlines your silhouette should stay on the rack; a slightly flared A-line will add length, not width, to your body.

A Touch of Scrawn

While flab is aging, the loose-and-skinny look won't subtract 10 years from your look either. If you have scrawny upper arms and inner thighs, the weight-training lifts for these areas outlined above will give you a firmer (therefore shapelier) look. If you're bothered by "crane legs," skinny calves supporting a more-than-size-8 body, add this exercise to your fill-out routine:

℞ FOR CRANE LEGS:

With ankle weights in place, stand barefoot, feet about 6 inches apart, toes pointing forward, arms gripping the back of a straight chair for balance. Rise on tiptoes, hold for 3 seconds, and lower your body (keep spine straight throughout) into a deep knee bend, still on tiptoe. Repeat, rising on tiptoes followed by knee bend 10 times, and watch your calves develop some necessary muscle.

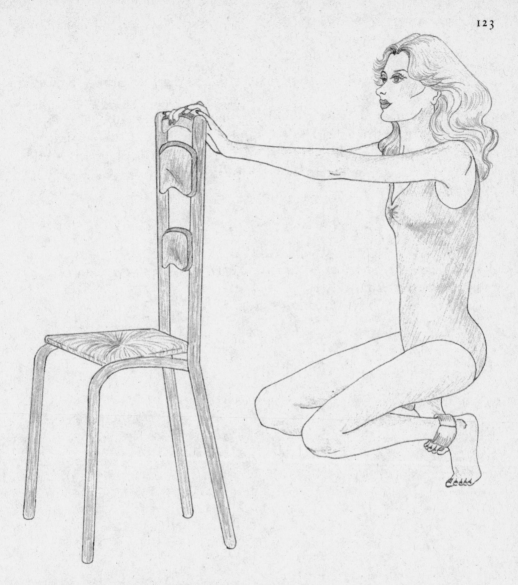

℞ TO CAMOUFLAGE CRANE LEGS:

Don't wear very billowing skirts; the contrast with your "meatless" calves will be overwhelming. Slightly tailored skirts or skirts/dresses that aren't very full at the hemline will work.

Try patterned or textured stockings, in a light or neutral color.

Boots that cover your calves are a natural.

Avoid clunky shoes, ankle straps. Simple shoes without crisscrossing work best.

℞ TO TIGHTEN INNER THIGHS:

Strap on ankle weights, lie on back with legs together, arms extended at sides. Curl knees over chest, then raise legs, feet flexed, toes pointing toward ceiling. Separate legs as wide as possible, trying to keep legs straight (position 1). Then bring legs together and cross right leg in front of left (position 2). Open legs wide again and recross with left leg over right. Repeat this crisscross movement 10 times nonstop. (Don't be surprised if it takes you awhile to work up to 10!)

℞ TO CAMOUFLAGE LOOSE INNER THIGHS:

Don't wear clingy slacks.

Consign short shorts to your favorite 16-year-old—wear tennis dresses and golf skirts instead.

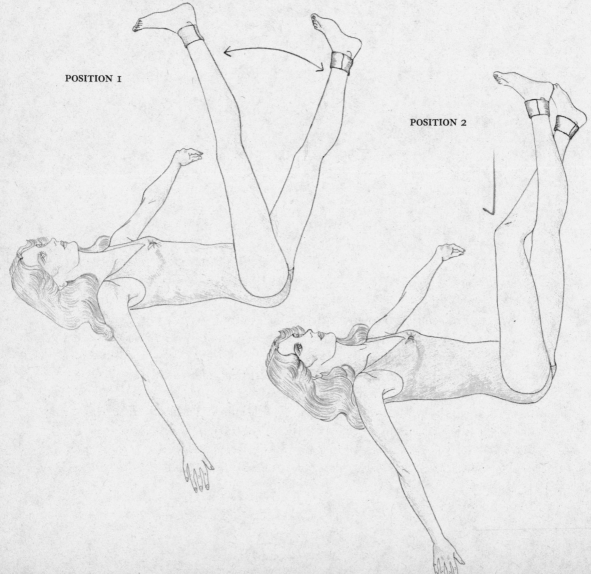

POSITION 1

POSITION 2

CHAPTER 9

❦❦❦

How to Look 10 Pounds Thinner,
10 Years Firmer
with Underwear Camouflage

The best now-you-see-it, now-you-don't magic will allow you to drop 10 years in 10 minutes and look 10 pounds thinner in the process. No, you needn't give your less than taut torso the evil eye. This no-trick solution simply involves choosing and using the variety of undergarments that the body engineers at the underwear firms have designed to firm up our bodies and help us look 10 years *better*.

I can't understand why a woman would take the time and trouble to exercise diligently and curb her calorie intake to the point where she's either *snarling* (at any poor soul who happens to say "have a nice day") or *salivating* (stealing an ice cream cone from a passing toddler is definitely considered anti-social behavior) when she actually can reproportion, smooth, lift, and firm her body, without lifting much more than a finger to sign her charge card, after she's been fitted for the correct undergarment.

While a trip to the lingerie specialty shop or intimate apparel section of a good department store won't be as mentally uplifting as an afternoon spent rereading *War and Peace* (in Russian, of course), there are times when it is more important to uplift your body (and soul) than your intellect.

That is why I want to take you inside the fitting room and behind the counter, to give you the knowledge that the store underwear buyers learn on the job. Consider what follows your body consciousness/camouflage training.

THE BRA PRIMER

The possibility of being asked to pose nude for a magazine centerfold decreases proportionately as your breasts begin to fall. And fall they will. Small breasts will tumble less than the larger variety, but it's an inevitable fact of life that gravity and age tend to weaken the support muscles somewhat and cause a bit of droop. However, because the breast itself is made up of soft fat and glandular tissue, *it can be uplifted, molded, rearranged, and repositioned.* . . . So what goes down can be brought back up.

What *type* of bra should you wear? It depends on your breast size and shape, of course—but it also depends on the clothes you favor. There is no such thing as the one right bra for you. You really need a bra wardrobe—different styles to give your bosom its best look under clingy clothes, low-cut or scoop necks, silky fabrics, and so on. So you must choose your bras to match your body *and* enhance your fashion image.

There are two basic ways to categorize bras, depending on the way they're constructed. First, you can choose either *seamless* or *cut-and-sew*—trade talk for seamed. Bras are also described according to what (besides you) goes into the cup—in other words, *type of padding*. Your bosom size and shape will dictate the construction details you need.

For Small to Average Bosoms

Seams vs. seamless isn't critical for you. What counts is the inside story, and what goes inside the cup is lining or padding.

A *thin layer of polyester fiberfill* just lines the cup so your nipple won't show through, and it gives a smooth, natural look to your bust. It also helps, if your flesh is less than self-supporting, by adding that layer of firmness you no longer have. If your breasts are slightly uneven, this bra will even you out (though it won't fill you out). If you're normal-sized but no longer 18-years-old firm, you may want this extra help.

A *contour bra* adds a little more fiberfill to help fill you out. If you're between an A and a B, for example, this bra will help you avoid the pleated-cup look. If your breasts have emptied from dieting, the contouring will take up the slack and still leave you with a natural line.

If you've become smaller as you've matured (I have often heard post-baby breasts referred to as "fried eggs"), check out the *padded bras*. The new padding (made of fiberfill or polyurethane foam) is designed *not* to bounce off the walls or invert (those of you who wore padded bras in high school may remember the fear your "breasts" would invert when dancing close!). Today's fully padded bra will jump you up one complete bra size without making you look as if you stepped into someone else's body. You try it on in the size you are, not the size you want to be.

If you're small or medium-sized and feel you need a little extra boost, try a seamless underwire. There are many versions, ranging from soft cup (no padding) up to fully padded. I wear a soft underwire bra with open shirts or low-cut blouses or dresses. It gives a slight pick-up without an obvious push. (If you're *average plus*, an underwire, *seamed* bra can give new definition to your silhouette.)

For Average to Large Bosoms

Seamed bras give more support because they are so designed that the seams act like built-in shapers. They are one good solution if you are not that big but have tended to hang a bit with the passage of time. They are absolutely necessary if you are large busted (no seamless knits for you) or have made the transition from slight sag to pendulous.

If you're becoming matronly large, ask for a "minimizer." Clever construction (usually with underwires) takes up to one inch off the amount the bust protrudes in front. When you put lots of flesh into the minimizer's

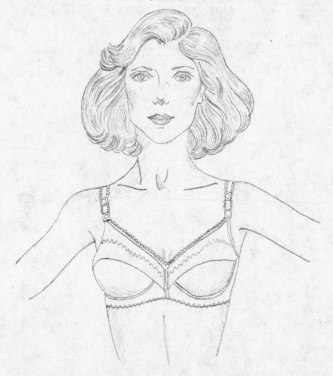

underwired cup, the wire flattens a bit, pulling tissue out to the side (it has to go somewhere!). The result is a sleeker look, especially good if your blouse button always looks as if it's ready to pop open over your cleavage. Make sure there's good cup separation, too. You want to look as though you have two separate and equal breasts, not one gigantic mass of glandular tissue.

You'll also want a bra with a wider strap to avoid an indentation mark in the shoulder caused by the heavy weight of the bosom.

Now you have an idea what to look for in seaming and/or padding. Here, some of the styles to fit your wardrobe and flatter your bustline:

Molded-cup bra: seamless bra, can be your everyday bra if you're small or medium-sized. Can be bought with or without fiberfill or underwiring. Works perfectly under sweaters because the no-seam, no-decoration look means no bumps under clingy clothes.

Front-closure bra: available in many cup styles, important if you wear clinging clothes (hooks poking out in the back of your sexy jersey break the line, look sloppy).

Demi-cup bra: wide-set straps and deep-plunging front make this the style for scoop neck and/or plunging necklines.

Push-up bra: so-called when bottom half of the demi-cup is lightly padded for push-up effect; many "demis" also feature underwire for yet more shaping and cleavage.

When wearing a push-up, assure *gentle* uplift by keeping the shoulder

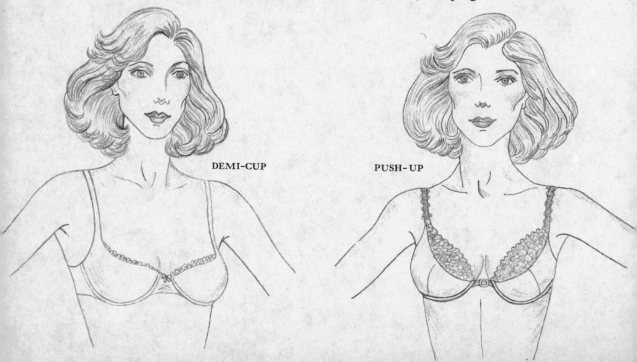

DEMI-CUP   PUSH-UP

straps comfortably firm. If you hike up your straps, you'll wind up with a Daisy Mae look, which isn't very contemporary.

The soft push-up cannot be worn under everything. Do not wear with a sweater or high-necked, clingy fabric. This bra only works with a low neckline or man-tailored shirt you wear with a button open to highlight your cleavage.

Halter-convertible bra: to wear with a halter top or dress if the back is bare and you don't want to go braless (if you're over 30, the braless look is not for you; even if you're small, you want to support your breasts to prevent early sagging). These bras are called "convertible" because they can be changed from halter style to one that crisscrosses in the back.

Strapless bras: for bare dresses. Since you'll be wearing this with sexy clothes, don't indulge in overkill by buying a strapless that allows you to overflow your dress. Your attempt to look like a Middle Ages serving wench will be middle-aging.

Foam inserts: pads that come in full- or half-cup styles. They give you that full and sexy look by creating additional cleavage. Place the inserts in your regular bra (in undercup, near armpits); the new snug fit will force your breasts together, give you a voluptuous look even if you're small. These are also terrific under a bathing suit. (Note: Give pads a trial run. Walk around with them for a while, swinging your arms about to make sure inserts are securely in place. If you bend over and foam falls into his soup, the color draining from your complexion will add 10 years to your looks!)

Two to Avoid

The "no-bra" bra: If you're in your 30s, you've probably worn this one. Seamless, underwireless, usually nude, made of the thinnest tricot (knit). These flimsy little styles are fine if you're a) very young, b) very firm, c) very small. If you're not two of these three, look for a bra that offers more support (you don't need a harness—but you may want a seamless with an underwire or a bit of fiberfill in a more supportive knit fabric, or a seamed style instead).

The one-size-fits-all bra: I'm sure there is a law of physics (if there isn't there should be) that states that matter can only be stretched so far. You want a bra that is proportioned to fit your true size; if it comfortably fits an A cup, the C-sized woman is bound to feel a bit uncomfortable and vice versa.

Fitting and Other Fundamentals

Knowing all about bra styles is just the beginning. Here, purchasing points to assure the bra you bring home is the bra you need.

℞. *Study your body proportions before you head for the lingerie department.* Example: Even though you're content with your bosom, it may not match up properly with your larger hips. If a body slimmer (trade talk for lightweight control garment—the heavy, boned girdle has gone the way of the dinosaur) alone won't bring you into proportion, you may want to try a lightly padded bra. If your bosom is large and you have just begun to sag, mention your problem to the saleswoman. The more you tell the fitter, the better chance that she will know how you want to look and be able to give you the bra et cetera that will fill your need.

℞. *Know just where your bosom should rest.* Of course, you don't want it to sag, but neither do you want to wear a bra that positions your nipples up at neck level. *With your bra on, the fullest part of your bust should rest even with an invisible point midway between your elbow and shoulder.* If yours is hovering lower, you are adding 10 years to your body image.

℞. *There really is only one correct way to put on a bra.* Slip straps over your shoulders, bend from the waist, let breasts fill cups, stand up, and attach hooks behind you. If you can't accomplish this maneuver, make front-hooking bras your wardrobe staple.

℞. *Get yourself a proper fit.* Many women don't know what size they truly are, so it's not wise to pick a few 34Bs (the most common size) off the rack and head for the checkout counter. When it comes to bras, my philosophy is the same as for make-up: I believe in *try before you buy*. In a good bra department or shop the saleswoman is trained to fit you, so let her take a few minutes with the tape measure.

You feel your local bra seller isn't a topnotch fitter? Fitting a bra is an art, and some customers bemoan the fact that the trained fitters of yesterday (those competent-looking women with tape measure slung around their necks, eyeglasses dangling from a chain, who take one look at you and say, "36C, of course, but let's just step into the fitting room to be sure, dear") *are* getting harder to find.

To make sure you and the saleswoman are on the same wavelength, determine your approximate size before you shop. The experts at Maidenform offer the following fit guide: Start by measuring your rib cage directly under your breasts. (Be sure to pull the tape snugly.) If the tape registers an odd number, add five inches, and the total will be your chest size. (You're 29 inches around? Add 5 inches. Now you know you wear a 34.) If you're an even number, add 4 inches (28 + 4 = size 32).

To get your cup size, let the tape rest comfortably as you measure around your back and across the fullest part of the bust (over your nipples). If your bust size is 1 inch larger than your adjusted body size, you're an A (i.e., your rib cage is 29, plus 5, or 34; your breast tissue measures 35, so you're a 34A); 2 inches greater, you're a B; $+ 3 = C; + 4 = D$.

℞. *Knowing your approximate size helps*, but there are so many fitting variables (your measuring skill, for one) that your reading of the Tale of the Tape shouldn't necessarily be considered the last word. If a saleswoman takes the time and trouble to suggest you're a different size and style from what you think, try on what she offers before you make a final decision. You may be the same weight and height you were when you were 18, but the 36B that cupped your breasts then might no longer do the best job if you're now sagging a bit or your breasts have changed shape.

℞. *Your bra is a misfit if:* flesh bulges over the top . . . bra cuts into underarm . . . undercup band doesn't hug rib cage (or hugs too tightly) . . . back rides up.

℞. *Take a twice-yearly trek to the lingerie department* to update your underwear wardrobe with new designs. If you find a shop you like, become a regular customer and ask them to let you know when manufacturers are sending in their traveling specialists. Then you can take part in a fitting clinic (very popular with customers) and learn what's new in the line while benefiting from the expertise of the best sizers in the business.

℞. *Experiment.* Just because you've always been comfortable with one bra style or one manufacturer, you (and your bustline) may be missing a lot of different enhancers. When you go on your next bra trip, take the time to try on a variety from different manufacturers.

℞. *Dress for the job.* When shopping for your everyday bras, wear a clinging sweater or silk shirt that will show everything; put your top back on after you try on each bra and study yourself in profile as well as head-on. The bra that looks terrific solo may not work so well under clothes.

Example A: If a bra gives you a too-pointy silhouette, you will look like Veronica from Archie comics—an old (not to mention aging) look. Example B: If your bra is too loose, it will show as a lumpy piece of cloth under your sweater. Example C: If the bra is too tight, you will look as though you have four breasts! You will also look the way you feel: uncomfortable. A bra that's tight is like shoes that pinch. Both make you look—and feel—grim.

℞. *Beware of lacy or highly decorated bras.* While these look wonderful in the bedroom, they may give you a bumpy, uneven look when you're dressed. A bra should not be visible under clothes.

℞. *Check out the way the straps look under clothes—front and back.* If you pull your straps too tight, you will produce a roll along the top in back and an indentation across the shoulders that will make your arms and chest look flabby even if they're not. If your straps are too loose, you'll always have to reach inside your shirt (like Ernestine, the holdover-from-the-1930s telephone operator created by comedienne Lily Tomlin) to hike them back up.

℞. *Keep the line in back as low as possible.* And as noted, for your clinging fabric dresses and tops, get a bra that hooks in the front. Speaking of back hooks, the properly fitting bra fastens at the tightest or next to tightest hook for a proper fit.

℞. *If you're choosing a bra for a special occasion outfit*, don't guess, bring the dress. It's the only way to make sure your bra will plunge as much as your neckline, your straps won't show, et cetera. When you buy your special dress, head for the bra department before heading for the exit and save yourself a return trip to the store.

℞. *If you run,* consider a good bra as important an investment as a pair of Pumas or Adidas. While running helps your cardiovascular system and your legs, it has a negative effect on the bosom. All that bouncing puts breasts under pressure, can lead to tissue breakdown (also known as sag). You want a bra that gives support, is made of an absorbent material like cotton, and has a wide underband to help keep it from riding up. Even if you're a firm A cup, wear a bra: Some joggers report bleeding from the nipples caused by the friction of breasts rubbing against a shirt. In fact, make a support bra *de rigueur* if you're engaging in any athletic endeavor.

THE BODY SLIMMER

The word "girdle" is becoming obsolete, and so is the type of garment it refers to: a multizippered steel-boned contraption complete with built-in garters that is so stiff it stands firmly at attention even when you're not wearing it. (Could this be what admen meant when they coined the slogan "living girdle"?)

Because these modern torture chambers rivaled the rack in their unsubtle attempts to change the human form, most women abandoned the girdle back in the 1960s and have worn no controllers since. But the opposite extreme, the let-it-all-hang-out look, is not only *unflattering* to most of us who are now less than completely firm (as in *unfirm*, not infirm), it is also *unnecessary*.

True, the heavy, uncomfortable underwear-of-the-damned styles are still available for those stalwarts who grew up with (and in) them, but for the rest of us who wouldn't be caught dead in a girdle, there are finally wearable alternatives based on the philosophy of comfortable yet chic cling first promoted by dance and swimwear makers.

This new generation of body slimmers works to hold us in and reshape us *naturally*. The result: a firmer-looking, inches-smaller silhouette.

Who needs what many manufacturers now call a body slimmer (other names: firmer/trimmer/smoother)? Most every woman over the age of 30 could use a little control for a sleeker look. You can have a terrific figure and still be plagued by a slight pot belly, dimpled outer thighs, drooping derrière (all problems unknown to a 16-year-old). Or, let's face it, you can have a truly less than terrific body and need more control to camouflage your problems, in which case the body slimmer will be an integral part of your everyday wardrobe.

Here, things to know and do before you buy:

℞. *Study the garment.* Today's slimmers firm and hold by using lightweight controlling fabrics like nylon and spandex (Lycra is Du Pont's trademarked name for the latter) and/or specially stitched knit and woven panels. The more spandex and paneling, the greater the control.

A nonpaneled slimmer will firm you, thanks to the controlling fabric, but it offers less pulling-in than the paneled variety. The placement of the panels indicates what figure problem the slimmer is designed to correct: stomach panels flatten abdomen, hip panels pull in hips, et cetera.

℞. *Buy the lightest, least constructed garment that works for you.* You want a little help to firm you up, but only where necessary—why pay for and wear panty legs, for example, when your tummy is the only trouble spot noticeable under clothes?

℞. *Try before you buy.* You must be fitted for your body slimmers with the same care you use to choose bras. Study your body so you can explain to the saleswoman what problem you want to camouflage. Do you need all-over firming? Are your thighs too fleshy? There are so many types of slimmer available, you'll want to match the solution to your own flaws.

℞. *Know your waist and hip dimensions* (measure hips at fullest point: 7 inches below your natural waistline). While manufacturers' sizing standards vary, at least you'll have an idea how you size up (medium is generally considered to fall between 37- and 40-inch hips).

℞. *Your slimmer fits if* 1) the waistline fits smoothly without pinching; 2) the crotch of the garment fits your natural crotch line—it shouldn't be too short, neither should it hang; 3) there's no bulge where the garment ends and your bare thigh begins.

℞. *Before you leave the fitting room*, sit and stand to make sure the slimmer doesn't buckle at the waist, creep up the thigh, or dig into you anywhere.

℞. *Know how to put it on*. If you need a slimmer with "legs," fold it in half (top over bottom) and step into it, pulling it up halfway. Then pull up the rest of the way and smooth into place.

℞. *If it feels good*, try it on under clothes to see if it makes you look good. If you're buying a slimmer to firm you under clingy clothes, make sure lace and paneling don't show through. For body-hugging knits, it's better to sacrifice some of the pull-in effects of strategic paneling for a seamless no-show model.

℞. *If you have a flat or sagging derrière* (the behind submits to gravity as much as the bustline—and droop here can be unnecessarily aging), there are excellent controllers that also lift your bottom, giving you a youthful, rounded contour rather than an all-girdled-in shape. Look for a seam or shirring (i.e., a puckered seam) going up the center of the back from the crotch to the waist. This will help lift and define the buttocks. Still other styles have a panel at the bottom that works like two hands to cup and lift your rear. These little wonder workers can actually change the way you look in pants.

℞. *Waist afflicted with "love handles"* (that extra inch or so of flesh that hangs around your middle)? Look for a slimmer with a *collar*, a wide band designed to cinch in your waistline.

℞. *Consider the body stocking*. I wear mine under see-through or clingy clothes. These are excellent when you need a little firming up all over and you want to hold your breasts in place. Today's lightweight nylon/spandex knit garments have built-in (or should I say knitted in?) holding power, yet they don't make you look and feel as if you're in an iron maiden. You may want to buy one with convertible straps so you can wear it under a variety of clothes. The snap-crotch opening adds to comfort and convenience.

℞. *Do a 16-year-old a favor*. If your daughter, sister, young neighbor, is bothered by a bit of baby fat and has taken to wearing a body firmer on a daily basis, tell her she's asking for trouble in the future. The best way for a young girl or woman to insure a future flat stomach, for example, is to make stomach muscles themselves work to hold her in. If you start to let a girdle do all the work for you when you're in your teens, you will have little or no visible muscles 10 years later. So when you peel off your undergarment at the age of 35, your body won't drop a mere inch or two—it will creep floorward and begin to ooze down the stairs!

Body Slimmer Style Guide

Slimmers come in almost as many styles as there are female forms. Consider the following:

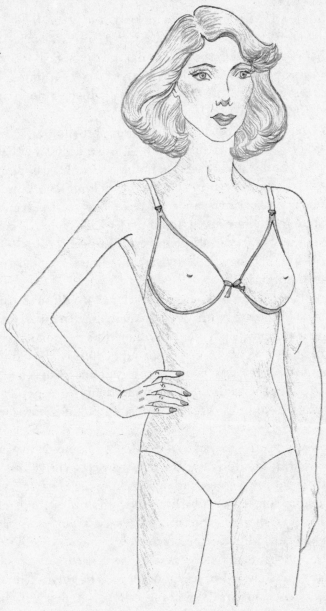

Brief: firms, molds, and controls from waist to the top of the thigh. The seamless, stretchy, no-panel variety is the most comfortable if you have no major problems and just need to be held in a bit. These also come with panels that slim specific problem areas, i.e., stomach, hips, buttocks. You can also get one in a derrière lift or French cut (high cut over the top of the thigh to expose more leg) style.

Sport brief: variation of the above, for the woman who would rather not jiggle on the tennis court. Lightweight, ventilated styling makes for comfort as well as control, yet allows maximum movability.

Panty leg: continues job of the brief by inching down the thigh. The newer ones are more comfortable because the clingy fabrics do the work and they don't have hooks for stockings that can dig into you. Still, I recommend them only as a measure of last resort. When you opt for almost total thigh coverage you are creating a stiff-looking body, which is not young-looking. (Firm is young; stiff is old.)

Instead, substitute support pantyhose. Today's support hose don't make you look as though you're encased in full-length Ace bandages; neither do they suggest feet shod in clunky black-laced grandma shoes. I wear the new sheer support hose quite often—they firm you up by holding everything in and they also help prevent varicosities and tired feet. They're indispensable if your job, like mine, requires you to stand on your feet a lot. Support pantyhose also keep you from looking as if all your flesh has been pushed down into a roll of less-than-firm flab dangling above your knees (which sometimes happens with panty leg girdles).

Hose-buying note: If you're a working woman who runs through pantyhose (whether support or regular) with budget-crunching frequency, you should know something about gauge and denier, which usually are marked on the hose package. Denier indicates fiber thickness, gauge refers to the closeness of the knit. If you're looking for durability, the *higher* the gauge and the *lower* the denier, the stronger the pantyhose (meaning they might not run or snag so easily . . . save the super-sheer and delicate stockings for special occasions).

Pant liner: smooths you from waist to mid-calf. These lightweight garments can give you a firm, slim look under dressy, flowing silk pants. For clingy, pencil-thin pants, choose a liner without side seams, then try your slacks over it. If the liner is thick, like a bathing suit, your slacks will cling to it and you may look as though you're wearing two pairs of pants! Elasticized cuffs help keep newer liners from creeping upward.

The "girdle-girdle": almost completely paneled for all-around maximum coverage; generally has garters instead of legs. Forget it! The totally encased, immobile look and feel will not only make you feel overcorseted, it will make your body look over the hill.

PANTIES

While some panties do contain spandex, they really don't offer much in the way of control. Still, the style you choose can help determine whether you look sleek or bulky.

Bikinis: the sexiest cut, can also be the unkindest if you have flesh overhanging the sides or a loose tummy.

Hip-huggers: a still-sexy alternative if your overhang is minimal. Choose one with a wide yet flat lace band around the top for a bit of extra camouflage.

Briefs: work best if you have something to hide (whether a bit of flab or stretch marks—you might as well keep the illusion going as long as possible), especially if they contain spandex or are of a stretchy material that will hold you in somewhat. Choose a satiny-looking brief with a French (high-cut) leg and you'll feel good (comfortable yet sexy) in them.

(*Slacks Caveat:* Even if you're a size 8, don't wear bikinis or hip-huggers under clinging or straight-legged pants. You'll have a cleaner, more bulge-free line if you wear waist-high briefs and pantyhose with built-in panties.)

Tap-pants (no elastic around the thighs): good if your legs tend to chafe as you walk. Today these are satiny and lacy, so you won't feel as if you're dressing to go ten rounds with Muhammad Ali. Of course, you can't wear "taps" under slacks or clingy clothes—and there's no point in stuffing them into a slimmer.

Speaking of stuffing, don't push your sweater or blouse inside your panties unless you're aiming for a thick-middled, misshapen look.

It doesn't hurt to try on underpants, either . . . and study yourself from the *back*. There's nothing more unflattering (or aging) than the sight of a dimpled behind hanging out the rear of underpants whose every line is showing through slacks or a clingy dress.

If you want to improve your rear view still further, underpants as well as slimmers come with a derrière-defining seam up the back—check out this style for another small (but every little bit helps!) behind booster.

No matter what style you choose, even if it's the teeniest bikini, insist upon a cotton crotch for comfort and hygiene.

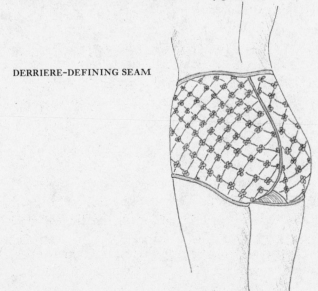

DERRIERE-DEFINING SEAM

THAT OLD BLACK (WHITE, NUDE) MAGIC: COLOR CUES

Bras, underpants, and slips come in devastating colors and patterns that can make you feel like a tigress underneath your gray flannel suit. Yes, you should indulge in a variety of stimulating colors and patterns, but make the backbone of your underwear collection *nude*. The tiger-stripe bra that looks so marvelous in the try-on room will make you look as though you're on the prowl if it shows through your sheers or thin knits, while practical nude goes under everything and shows under nothing.

The one underwear color you can safely eliminate from your wardrobe is *white*. Manufacturers say that the nude tones now sell equally with or better than white—for good reason. Not only does white turn gray and lifeless after repeated washings (and you remember what mother said about wearing clean underwear in case you're in an accident . . . how come mothers never suggest nice underwear in case you have a spur-of-the-moment chance for a brief encounter?), it also shows through under thin or lightweight fabrics.

Of course, women cannot buy underthings for practicality alone. The sensible nude I've just touted may make your body look a bit anemic, and probably won't set his pulse racing. If you want to make a dramatic statement when you take your clothes off, wear lace-trimmed red. Men are not very subtle, and though you think dusky mauve and teal blue look lovely, siren red still signals (in this case go, not stop) sex. Generally men go for deep colors that contrast with light skin.

When it comes to caring for intimate apparel, a little hand work will help delicates go a long way. Even if the hang tag says machine washable, don't use machines to wash and dry bras (especially underwires) and slimmers. I personally love silk underwear, but these must be hand washed *and ironed*, so they really aren't very practical.

NIGHT GAMES: HOW TO DRESS FOR BED

If you still have the body of a 19-year-old, you probably look terrific in a short, well-worn T-shirt with "Shazam" blazed across the front.

But if you're a mere mortal like the rest of us, you should give a little thought to the way you dress for bed. Pretty nightgowns that help you feel good about your body will help you enjoy sex more . . . and a satisfying sex life is definitely a part of looking 10 years younger.

Even if you've shared the same bed with the same man for years (or if it only seems like years!), giving some thought to choosing your nightwear is just as important as the care you invest in buying a good suit or dress.

Looking good when I go to bed makes me feel sexy. I keep on my mascara, for example, because I just don't like the pale-lashed, less-dramatic-eyed look I have without it. And why should my night image differ from the self I've created for day?

Luckily for those of us who can no longer get away with the baby-doll look but have no desire to succumb to a flannel granny gown, there are alternatives that will help transmit high-voltage bedroom glamour. Remember, a little mystery combined with a length of sheer, satiny fabric is more of a turn-on than jumping into the bedroom clad in a smile and the Emperor's new clothes (you wouldn't have caught the Empress framed in the doorway in the altogether—not if she were over 25).

There are decidedly sexy gowns that will wrap you in intrigue and sophistication and make you look and *feel* like the body beautiful, which is half the battle. Even the flimsiest nightdress has features that can make (or break) your body. So shop with a sharp eye toward *revealing* camouflage (no, that's not a contradiction) and you'll be ready to play to win in the bedroom.

Is a healthy preoccupation with creating an aura of glamour unliberated? Only to those who think a healthy preoccupation with sex is unliberated. If dressing for bed makes you feel ready for bed, do it—and don't apologize.

Consider the following night dressing suggestions:

℞. *Go wild with deep, body-contrasting colors.* You're in the bedroom anyway; why not be blatant? Save pale pink and baby blue for your trip to the maternity ward or your post-appendectomy recuperation.

℞. *Reveal your hidden image via nightwear.* If you're a super-efficient executive by day, satin and lace, provocatively cut, will show a new side of your personality that it would be inappropriate (to say the least) to display around the office.

℞. *If you're small-breasted,* look for gowns that come with a built-in lightly fiberfilled bra section, and invest in soft lighting.

℞. *Make a small bust appear larger* by choosing a bodice that's shirred, laced, printed, highly designed . . . or a gown with a drawstring under the bust that you can tie tightly to create a little cleavage.

℞. *If you're really flat-chested,* don't wear a deeply plunging neckline; instead, choose a high neck and add drama with a deep plunge that shows off your back.

℞. *If you're matronly large,* buy a gown with a built-in unpadded bra for support.

℞. *A stretchy-topped gown* will help hold you in and up if you're a bit large.

℞. *An Empire-style gown* (especially paired with an elasticized high waistband) can give you some built-in pick-up if you're starting to hang a bit.

℞. *To camouflage a few extra pounds*, buy a float—a caftan-style gown that floats seamless and tuckless down from the shoulders to the floor. It will swirl around (rather than pull around) your body in a most becoming way.

℞. *Emphasize a small waist* by buying a gown with a fitted waistband; deemphasize a large waist by buying a blouson style (yes, they do make them).

℞. *Darts that end under the bust* call attention to this feature.

℞. *Thin spaghetti straps* show off smooth throat, gleaming shoulders.

℞. *Some gowns are elasticized across the back*—good if you have a little roll of fat behind your waist, across your midriff.

℞. *A short teddy with a covered camisole top* will look terrific if your legs are your best feature.

℞. *If you like the leggy look of a teddy or baby doll* but your body is no longer total perfection, there are gowns that open down the front, matched with bikini bottoms. The gown will flow over your silhouette, hiding less than firm outer thighs or widening hips . . . yet the bare front will give you a sexy, bikinied look.

❧❧❧

PART FIVE

HAIR:
IT DOESN'T
WRINKLE,
BUT IT AGES

CHAPTER 10

❧❧❧

Everything You Need to Know to Correct Hair That's Gone from Wash-and-Wear to Washed-Out and Worn

Are you still a virgin?

No, it's not your bedroom activity that interests me—it's your hair, and what you do to (and for) it. Virgin hair is unprocessed and practically untouched by human or mechanical hands—hair that has never known anything but the innocent caress of shampoo, comb, and brush.

You do possess virgin hair, and are proud of your purity? Don't be too smug—if you're 30ish, your "I was born this way" hair is definitely starting to age, probably starting to fade, and quite likely beginning to look a bit drab. (After all, there's nothing more dull, listless, and boring than an old virgin!) To correct drab hair, you have to step over the brink and submit your head to some life-giving, luster-adding activities. A bit of judicious treatment will give dull hair a 10-years-younger lift, and young hair makes everything else about you look more alive, whereas faded hair can make you look as though you're content to spend your days darning socks and your nights knitting afghans for a single (rather than king-sized) bed.

You say you've never been satisfied to leave your hair alone? You say you've *done it all*—twisted your hair into more different styles than the *Joy of Sex* has positions, been indiscriminate with hair color since you first discovered peroxide in the corner drugstore, haven't felt your hair's natural texture since you wore bobby sox? If so, you hair undoubtedly looks played out, fizzed and frazzled out, and generally over the hill.

Well, step right up and let me show you the road to salvation.

Luckily for all of us, hair is one part of the anatomy that can be reversed to a born-again state of *better* than virginal innocence.

Whether you're promiscuous or virginal or middle of the road so far as your hair goes, it will begin to collapse, along with your spirits, as you reach your 30ish birthday. But there's really no need for "I can't stand my hair!" depression (there are plenty of more important reasons to be depressed). If you have the proper hair facts, you can possess swinging, shiny, healthy-looking hair. So stop yanking out those first gray hairs or counting the strands in your brush, and start reading.

THE SUBJECT IN QUESTION

Hair, like Gaul, is divided into three parts.

The *medulla*, or innermost part of the hair shaft, does Lord knows what. Scientists still aren't sure of its function. In fact, if you have thin hair (in the sense that the diameter of each strand is thinner than average, not meaning thin in the sense you're losing some of what you've got), you may not have a medulla at all.

The mysteries of the middle (and largest) layer, the *cortex*, have been solved. The pigments responsible for your hair color are located in the middle "C"; the cortex is the part most affected when you color your hair.

The *cuticle*, or outermost layer, is the most important if healthy, shiny hair is your goal. It protects the cortex from the ravages of the environment and locks moisture within the hair shaft. (Hair, like skin, is made of a form of protein called keratin. And like skin, it needs oil and moisture to stay healthy.) A cuticle has layers like an artichoke's. If the layers are raised and open (because of dryness or damage), the cuticle won't lie flat. Who cares? *You should*. Light is reflected off a flat smooth surface as shine. I'll explain how to close and flatten your cuticle shortly.

The hair you love to touch is *dead*. The only living parts of the hair apparatus are the parts you don't see. Each individual hair grows out of its own follicle embedded in the scalp; each follicle is fed by its own papilla, which in turn is nourished by capillaries that transmit nutrients carried by your blood. This is why good scalp circulation is as important as good skin circulation. Equally crucial for lush locks: a good diet (your hair is only as healthy as the "food" carried to it by the blood).

Though your crowning glory is technically dead, you won't be accused of being a necrophiliac if you try to bring it back to what looks like glowing life. Nor need you be Harry Houdini to correct many of the hair problems most of us are heir to as we get older. The best way I can start helping your hair escape from the bonds of drabness and damage is to throw open the notebooks I bring to beauty seminars and answer for you the questions I'm most frequently asked.

HOW TO REV UP "3-D" HAIR

One look at my once crowning glory and heads turn—in the opposite direction. My hair suffers from the 3 Ds—it's dull, drab, dead-looking. How come?

Any of four main problems could be causing your "3-D" hair.

Possibility #1: Age

Your hair could be getting drab because of age. "Senile" hair—faded, dull, a mere ghost of its former vibrant self—can start creeping up on us when we're in our late 20s, early 30s—mere babes by gerontological standards. The hair color pigments (or melanin) housed in the cortex stage a slowdown, leading to faded hair. Eventually they go on a permanent strike, leading to no-color (or gray) hair. Loss of pigment is influenced by a built-in time clock in the follicles. Ask your parents when their gray hair punched in and you'll know what to expect. If your hair looks drab because the color is fading and gray shoots are sprouting up, check out "First Gray and Other Sorrows," Chapter 12.

Possibility #2: Abuse or Neglect

If you hair color hasn't grayed or faded, your hair could look dull because of abuse or neglect. It may lack shine because the outermost layer, the cuticle, has been "pried open" by too much processing and too little conditioning. An open cuticle results when hair is overbleached or overpermed, making it porous, but not treated with conditioners to reclose the cuticle. The cuticle must not only lie flat and smooth (to reflect light), it must also be tightly closed (to seal in the natural oils your scalp supplies).

Possibility #3: Improper Regimen

You could be the possessor of "3-D" hair simply because you're using the wrong wash and care products. Hair, like skin, starts to dry out as birthdays add up, and just as you must change your face-treatment routine to compensate, so should your hair-care schedule be updated. Check the wash and care guide, pages 156–61.

Possibility #4: Improper Feeding

Your dull, prematurely faded, and dead-looking hair could be the result of improper feeding. In other words, your follicles aren't getting the nourishment they need to produce a shiny, swinging mane. You can condition your hair from here to St. Swithin's Day, but if you're not getting an adequate diet, don't expect your hair to roll over and look alive. Fortunately, what's crucial to 10-years-younger hair also makes sense for good general health. I asked Dr. Klein, whom you met in the diet chapter, to gear his nutritional know-how to the in-between woman who wants to produce a good crop of hair.

Dr. Klein's 10 Prescriptions for 10-Years-Younger Super Hair

℞ #1. *Stoke up on the B complex.* You may not have needed the B-boost when you were younger, but Dr. Klein says the B-plex vitamins are "the key to beautiful hair . . . they promote luxuriant hair growth and strengthen the hair shaft. Choline, inositol, and biotin are three components of the B complex important for continued hair growth, and along with PABA and pantothenic acid they may help prevent the appearance of prematurely gray hair." Dr. K. says you can ingest up to 150 mg of PABA daily, but if you take one particular B, you must make sure you're also taking the whole complex in adjusted proportions to avoid an imbalance. It's OK for Dr. Klein to split his Bs—he's a doctor of nutrition; but to avoid health complications, don't make it a habit to play around with your Bs without professional advice. I just swallow the richest complex I can buy, except when I'm taking my anti-stress Dracula drink for just a few days. A good B capsule will contain 50 mg of B_1, B_2, B_6, niacin, biotin; 50 mcg B_{12}; 1,000 mcg folic acid.

℞ #2. *Avoid the B depleters.* Alcohol, caffeine, sugar, stress, starches. The birth control pill is yet another B destroyer, so if you're on the Pill you should also hop on the B bandwagon.

℞ #3. *Avoid stress and other C depleters.* If it would be easier for you to stop breathing than to stop worrying, compensate by taking vitamin C. Besides impairing scalp circulation, stress can burn up 3,000 to 4,000 mg of vitamin C in a period of hours. Since C helps rebuild tissues (your hair and skin are both made of similar tissue substances—what's good/bad for skin is also good/bad for hair), it is important to hair production. C also helps detoxify the blood—and the better the state of your blood, the more efficiently it will transport nutrients to your scalp. Smoking, as I've mentioned previously, is a C depleter; so are aspirin, tobacco, and heat (refrigerate *all* vitamins). Dr. K. says the best way to get your C is via natural, time-released tablets (found in health food stores); 500 mg in the A.M., 500 mg in the P.M., is a good hair-repair dosage.

℞ #4. *Boost circulation to your scalp internally* by taking vitamin E. Start with 100 units a day; gradually work up to 400. E also makes an excellent scalp ointment. Break open capsules and massage into scalp and hair before you shampoo. (Note: If you have high blood pressure or other circulatory problems, don't take E internally without your doctor's approval.) Wheat germ, cold-pressed safflower oil, nuts, and grains are rich in E; taking the Pill depletes it.

℞ #5. *Too much vitamin D promotes temporary hair loss.* Stick with the doses provided in your multivitamin.

℞ #6. *Consider the hair minerals.* Zinc is essential for stronger hair shafts and more luxe growth; it also prevents fallout to some degree. Dr. K. says you can take up to 150 mg a day (more would be toxic) or find it in shellfish, spinach, brewer's yeast, sunflower seeds. Copper is the anti-gray mineral; take 3 or 4 mg a day, or find it in nuts, seafood, raisins. (Exception: If your drinking water flows through copper pipes, you may be getting more than your share of copper—check with your local water department.) You're not sure how much your hair (and body) requires? Find these minerals in a *multimineral supplement,* or better yet, have your doctor send a sample of your hair to a hair analysis center. Mineral deficiencies often show up in your hair before they become apparent in the rest of your body.

℞ #7. *Make sure you're not anemic.* Iron is another mineral essential to healthy hair growth. If you think you're lacking, ask your doctor to test you and prescribe iron supplements if necessary.

℞. #8. *Consider cold-pressed oil.* C.P.O. not only contains vitamin E, it also lubricates your hair, helping to prevent dryness and brittleness. If you have a pedigreed pooch, you can be sure your dog handler or veterinarian will insist you include oil in your dog's diet—it helps promote a glossy coat. Why not pamper your own hair as well? If your hair is dry, add one teaspoon of oil (the cold-pressed, unprocessed variety found in health food stores) to your daily diet.

℞ #9. *Eat plenty of protein,* 50 or 60 grams a day. Hair, keratin—call it what you will, it still spells protein, and a protein-deficient diet leads to old-looking, lifeless hair. Chicken, turkey, fish, veal, eggs, liver, low-fat milk, and low-fat cheese should be part of your intake.

℞ #10. *Reconnoiter the health food stores*, ask questions, and learn to eat like a nutritionist. You may have lived on the all-American hamburger-cola-fries diet as a kid, but you won't be unpatriotic if you switch your allegiance to beauty foods. If you're serious about having healthy, shining hair, it's time to learn to love brewer's yeast and desiccated liver for their B vitamins; grains, nuts, and seeds for vitamin E; and wheat germ for E and protein.

A FAT REPORT ON FIGHTING THINNING HAIR

I'd give a fortune to have "rich girl" hair—thick, luxurious locks that titled women with hyphenated names seem to possess forever. But at the tender age of 33, my hair, once adequate, is getting a bit thinner. Do you need blue blood to keep thick hair?

Her Ladyship Pamela Smedley-Smythe is on a first-name basis with the top hair doctors, trichologists (hair analysts found in top salons), haircutters, and nutritionists on four continents (I'm not sure *what* she does when she tours Antarctica!). And what these pros tell her helps her keep her hair looking voluminous from the cradle to the grave. You're now going to learn the "secrets" rich girls pay dearly for.

But first, we have to define our terms. At this point I'm not talking about fine hair, wherein, as mentioned, you were unlucky enough to be the hereditary victim of underweight hair genes (if that's your problem, stay tuned). Rather, I want to tell you what to do if your hair just doesn't seem as full as it used to, if you seem to be losing more than you'd like of what you've got.

Pregnancy and the Pill

Temporary hair loss can be caused by pregnancy. Your body is just too busy producing nourishment for the baby-to-be to worry about what's doing with your hair. That's why a few months after you take your first new-mother bows, when hair factory production starts making up for lost time, you may notice an inordinate amount of shedding. Not to worry. This hair loss is almost always temporary, as is fallout related to the Pill.

℞. *To cope, treat your hair gently* for the duration. Don't perm, color, overheat with appliances, brush 100 strokes. Give your hair a chance to return to health.

Booze and Tobacco

If you're neither pro nor con pregnancy, but you do smoke and/or drink, your hair may react by thinning while your skin is aging. Smoking is anti-hair because, as you now know (I'll turn you into a nutritionist yet), it robs the body of vitamin C, important for hair health, *and* narrows the blood vessels. Since blood is the messenger that carries nutrients to the follicles, *constricted* blood vessels mean less "food" is able to swim through the vessels to the papillae, where new hair is born.

Drinking is anti-hair because "demon rum" destroys the crucial B-for-Beautiful-Hair vitamins.

℞. *To cope, be conspicuous in your consumption* of the proper nutrients. If your food and vitamin intake doesn't somewhat parallel Dr. Klein's program, your hair probably isn't just dull—you may be encouraging thinning, which is discouraging.

Look to Your Nerves

Tension leads to telogen, or the stage during which hair falls out. About 85 percent of normal hair is in the anagen, or growth, stage and will stay firmly anchored to your scalp for two to six years. Some hair loss is to be expected. The remaining 15 percent of growth is old hair that is loosening and shedding to make way for new young hair—this falling telogen hair is what you see on your brush in the morning. But if you're overwhelmed by stress, tension, anxiety—that state of bad vibrations characterized by a tight feeling across your shoulders, up your neck, *and* into your scalp—your state of stress could be cutting off some needed circulation to the follicles. Trichologists, who work with microscopes and other modern gizmos to determine your hair health, call this the "tight scalp syndrome," and it may be causing your growth phase to stop dead in its tracks, and your telogen phase to continue unabated. The reason: Once again, constricted blood vessels, which go hair in hand with a tight scalp, keep adequate nourishment from reaching the hair bulb.

℞. *To cope, use a slantboard*. It will help relax you and stimulate the flow of blood to your head.

℞. *Unwind your tight scalp*. Hairologists, not to mention good old-fashioned hairdressers, stress the value of scalp massage to combat stress, which in turn will allow essential nutrients (you are eating right, taking the correct vitamins, aren't you?) to reach the papillae. Perform a scalp massage twice weekly. When you feel your scalp warm up and tingle, you know you've done the job properly.

Massage *won't* help you if you're going bald (when hair suddenly and dramatically starts falling out in great clumps, it's time to hotfoot it to the nearest dermatologist—hormonal changes or illness could be the cause). But massage will help you improve scalp circulation, which could be all the R you need if you've been under extreme tension and have been walking around wearing a scalp two sizes too small.

To properly de-tense your scalp, drop your head forward and place your open palms on your scalp underneath your hair. With short strokes, slide your fingertips (not nails) and palms from nape to crown in a push/relax series of movements. Now move your fingertips along your scalp in circular motions. Do you feel your scalp move and tingle? Does your head feel warm? If so, you've sufficiently loosened and de-kinked your tight scalp.

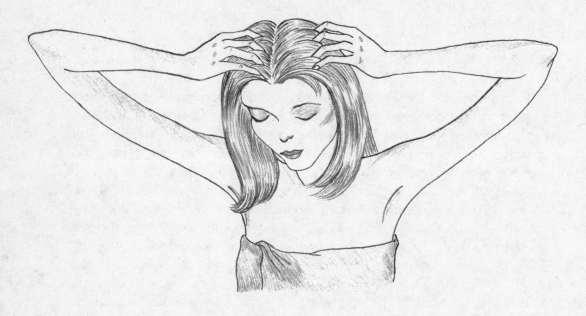

The Wages of Sin

If you've been perming, bleaching, and dyeing indiscriminately for years, without remorse *or* conditioners, and have a habit of absent-mindedly setting your blow dryer on "scorch" and keeping it in one place for several minutes, you don't have true thinning hair—rather, you have beaten-up hair, which resembles hair loss because the damaged hairs get brittle and break off close to the scalp before they have a chance really to grow. There's nothing wrong with the roots, papillae, follicles, yet you look as though you have hardly any hair at all.

℞. *To cope, show your hair some mercy.* You need a careful treatment regimen to bring your hair back to a young look from its present over-the-hill, much-abused state. I'll go into the products and procedures to take 10 years off the look of damaged hair as the chapter proceeds.

'Tis the Season

If you're shedding more and enjoying it less, check the calendar. Hair looks fuller in summer, because we lose fewer hairs then; one reason it looks thinner in winter is that we shed more during the cold weather. The greatest hair loss is reported to occur in the brisk month of November.

Loss of up to 100 hairs a day is normal (the average head contains about 100,000 hairs); more than 100 daily is considered excessive, and would make me a wee bit nervous if it continued over an extended period.

Blondes may not necessarily have more fun but they do have more hair —maybe to compensate for the fact that their individual hair shafts are thinner.

You should also know that if you still want hair halfway down your back, you probably can no longer have it. Hair grows longest between the ages of 15 and 30; once we hit 30, the whole anagen-telogen hair growth cycle starts to slow down, along with metabolism, nail growth, sebum production. This doesn't mean we fold up our beauty tents and go home; it just means we work a little harder to keep our hair looking as healthy as it did 10 years ago.

Study Your Scalp

If your scalp, whence all hair protrudes, is unhealthy, your hair could be thinning. Seborrhea, which looks to the lay person like a severe case of runaway dandruff, is an inflammation of the hair follicle that can be reversed by topical injections of steroids into the scalp. If your scalp looks less than normal, take yourself to a dermatologist.

Other assaults on the body can affect your head. High fever, trauma caused by an accident or surgery, are two possible causes of temporary hair loss. As you recuperate, so will your hair.

Bad Genes

While I'm sure "bad" blood and a tendency to lunacy don't run in your family as they do in those of Gothic heroines, you well may have inherited poor-quality hair. If mom, dad, and their forebears started thinning early, you're probably just following the unlucky pattern predetermined at your birth.

Dr. Hillard Pearlstein, assistant clinical professor of dermatology at Mount Sinai School of Medicine and Mount Sinai Hospital, New York City, implicates hormones along with heredity. As women age, we produce less estrogen so the effects of the male hormone androgen (which women also produce in small quantities) are more apparent. If your particular hair follicles are sensitive to the androgen you produce (and it's an inherited sensitivity), you may be in for some all-over permanent hair loss.

Androgen is the hormone associated with MPB (male pattern baldness). Could that be why bald men are considered virile?

You can't stop this natural, progressive hair loss, but you needn't worry that it will lead to the loss of all your hair. True baldness of the Telly Savalas and Yul Brynner variety is virtually nonexistent in women (as well as men) —the less obvious over-all thinning (which affects more women after menopause) can begin much earlier if your genes so determine.

℞. *To cope, minimize the problem* by treating hair gently both mechanically (no hot blow dryers, no vigorous toweling) and chemically (if you want a gentle perm or coloring, have it done professionally). Make it appear fuller by using the right wash and care products.

Equally important (and possible) is styling thinning hair to camouflage the problem. How-tos are in the next chapter.

I am considering seeing a dermatologist for my thinning hair. What can he/she do to—and for—me?

Dr. Pearlstein explains that the clues provided by *testing and talking* can often (not always) help the doctors diagnose the "whys" of premature fallout so appropriate treatment can be undertaken. If you have seborrhea, as mentioned, severe psoriasis, or other scalp disorders that are blocking the appearance of hair, the disease can often be cleared up—and with it, your fallout problem. Or you may be tested for thyroid deficiency, endocrine (hormonal) dysfunctions, or anemia. There are also tests that enable the physician to determine what percent of your follicles are in the anagen (growth) stage. It may be determined that you're just in a stepped-up shedding phase—and normal growth will return. It's better (though more depressing) to lose 150 hairs a day that will return than 5 hairs doomed never to come back.

The thorough doctor will also ask whether or not you've recently had a baby or abortion, are taking or have stopped taking the Pill, are on any special medication or following a severely restricted diet, have been twisting, over-brushing, or otherwise mechanically and chemically abusing your hair—all could affect the state of your locks.

If one area of your head looks particularly sparse, while growth else-where is OK, remember—your driver's license needn't be checked *male* for you to check out a transplant. Whether it's because women are under more stress than before (with career decisions adding to or substituting for the dif-ficult job of caring for a family), or are doing more to their hair now (blow dryers, curling irons, electric rollers, too frequent perms—I coud go on), the complaints of premature fallout are rising as our hair is thinning.

Here's how transplants work: Tiny plugs of scalp skin containing healthy follicles are transplanted to a thin spot, where they will once again produce healthy hairs. The number of visits you'll make to the dermatologist depends on how much transplanting you need done—often, the job can be completed in 3 or 4 visits, with up to 70 tiny plugs (each containing 10 to 15 hairs) transplanted per session. It takes about 4 months to see growth, 8 to 12 months for good long-haired results, but most transplantees feel the results eventually justify the wait. Remember, only a doctor can decide if your condition war-rants the treatment—and only a doctor should be entrusted with the task.

One final word: If two respected dermatologists (I always believe in a second opinion) tell you nothing can be done, if they firmly believe your thinning hair is caused by hereditary factors that can't be reversed, accept their verdict and buoy your spirits by remembering that only men go billiard-ball bald. Most of all, don't feel you have to buy out the stock of the local turban saleswoman. Instead, continue to nourish what hair you have via a healthy diet, proper supplements, gentle care, and effective cosmetic com-pensations (thickeners, cuts, styling, tinting—yes, proper coloring can help) that will make it obvious to you alone that you have a problem.

TO FATTEN FINE HAIR

I am semi-unfortunate. My hair is healthy, swingy, and bouncy, but (here's the unfortunate part) naturally fine. Now that my face is start-ing to lose its smooth, girlish charm, I think it's important to counter-balance my incipient crow's-feet with full hair. How do I fatten fine hair?

If you've maintained your hair in good health and are interested in a magic potion that will help you grow fatter hair strands, remember you've just opened a book, not rubbed a magic lantern or shouted "Open Sesame"! *What is genetically predetermined, no beauty expert can go back and undo.* But you can successfully create the *illusion* of fuller hair by using the right conditioners and thickeners (wonder workers I'll describe shortly) and by choosing a hairstyle that doesn't accentuate your hereditary "deficiency."

You can also color and curl your hair. Did you know that processing can actually be *good* for fine, healthy hair? The chemicals in single-process coloring tints and permanents are alkaline, so they make the cuticle stand away from the cortex, slightly enlarging the diameter of each hair shaft. Since your hair is healthy, you can indulge!

One more point: If your hallmark is still girlish charm, it's time to trade in the ingénue look for sophisticated glamour. As the new in-between woman, you no longer need to rely on young-girl innocence.

D-D-DANDRUFF

One back-to-work "benefit" I didn't count on is dandruff. I never had this problem before. Why now?

While stress can cause hair thinning in some people, *your* body may be responding to a newly tension-filled situation by producing scalp flaking. Nervousness causes the oil-producing glands to work overtime, which is further causing scalp cells to clump together and shed in bunches. In addition, if you're working in a modern, sealed office building, the air is probably very dry from central heating and air conditioning, and your scalp, like your skin, is drying out.

While you can't demand a humidifier for the office (not until you become chairperson of the board), you can install one at home for nighttime scalp and hair hydration as well as for skin moisturization. You should also take the time for a pre-shampoo scalp massage to help hurry the demise of the debris: massage sloughs your scalp to remove old dead cells just as sloughing helps your skin de-clump. Assuming your scalp trouble isn't accompanied by hair stress, thorough (but not rough) brushing will also speed recovery.

℞. *Use a dandruff shampoo* containing zinc, tar, sulfur, or selenium pyrithione once a week, until your scalp (and your nerves) calms down.

ENVIRONMENTAL IMPACT STUDY

My hair suddenly seems very sensitive to the environment. . . . Is this because I'm getting older?

No, you're just getting wiser! Hair, like skin, responds positively or negatively to what it's exposed to, and must be treated accordingly.

℞ *for sun*. Cover up your hair—especially if it's naturally dry, permed, or colored. Most people don't realize the sun fades *natural* as well as added color. Condition sun-dried hair more frequently. If you're sunbathing (hopefully, you're not), comb conditioner through hair beforehand—ditto if swimming in chlorinated water.

Plus for the sun: Your hair sheds less and it expands (swells) in hot, dry weather—so it looks fuller.

℞ *for heat and humidity*. Both increase perspiration and sebum production, so you'll have to wash your hair more often.

If your hair looks dry, shampoo gently. Even if the added washing is gentle, it may strip more natural oils from your hair than you'd like, so you must use an instant conditioner regularly.

If your hair looks oily, be sure that you use your all-purpose shampoo more frequently. Be sure also that you make your final rinse cold water to stop limpness. If you're in a humid climate, you also have to adapt your hairstyle to thrive in the "wet heat" phenomenon, which means getting a good cut that won't make you dependent on setting your hair each time you step out the door.

℞ *for the cold*. No matter what hair type you have, it will probably look its worst in winter. First, because winter is the shedding season, the added fallout makes your hair thinner. Second, the erector pili muscle housed beneath the follicle contracts in the cold, making hair hang limp, close to the scalp. To counteract these problems, plus winter dryness, you might want to add a weekly or monthly (depending on the state of your hair) deep conditioner to your care routine, and wear a scarf when you go outdoors. Covering your head does more than keep your ears warm—it also keeps hair from getting brittle, and brittleness can lead to split ends.

Winter is also static electricity season. The combination of dropping temperatures and dry air makes for flyaway hair. To moisturize normally textured or dry hair—and fight the flyaways—use a cream rinse even if you didn't need one in summer (the humidity in summer air creates a warm moisture coating for your hair); if your hair is oily but flyaway, a *diluted* cream rinse applied along the shaft away from the roots (where oil tends to congregate) will increase manageability without increasing limpness.

Cold, dry air can also lead to flaking scalp—a heavy-duty conditioning treatment weekly, plus the use of your trusty humidifier at night, will help clear the problem.

THE 10-YEARS-OFF WASH AND CARE SHOPPING GUIDE

🌀 *My hair used to thrive on a regimen of baby shampoo, boar's hair brush and blow dry. But the shine and body of yesteryear are no longer apparent. What do I put on my hair to make it look young and healthy again?*

Most drugstores stock more hair products than cold remedies. And while common cold research hasn't progressed much beyond the aspirin and vitamin C stage, that wealth of hair-correcting products really can make a life-or-death difference to your hair's appearance, if you know how and when to use them.

But you must be realistic about what they can and can't do. There is no treatment you can apply to the surface of the hair to make it grow thick and healthy, because as we have noted, hair is born below the scalp and is influenced by diet, nerves and heredity. The products I'm about to describe won't penetrate the scalp and its attendant follicular network, but it almost doesn't matter. Because if you're in good health, you *can* coat and/or penetrate the hair shaft with products that can help duplicate the look of young, lively hair.

Here's what you need to know to rejuvenate, if not regenerate, your hair.

SHAMPOO . . .

Shampoo has just one function: to cleanse the hair and scalp.

When you choose your shampoo, if you're tinting your hair, look for one whose label also reads color-fast. Almost all shampoos rely on detergents (which are alkaline) for their cleansing power, but if your hair is less than healthy, look for one that has ingredients that tilt the formula to an acid-balanced state (check the label). You don't have to worry about the acidity at all if your hair is normal.

You're worried because the manufacturer of the shampoo you love makes no pH claims? There's no need for an anxiety attack. No major shampoo brand marketed today is so alkaline that it's a hair destroyer.

Before you suds, de-tangle your hair with a comb, and massage your scalp.

If you think of your hair as a fabric, remember, you wash hair following the same principles as you use with laundry: the warmer the water, the cleaner the garment (or hair). Of course, you *don't* wash hair in *hot-hot* water (third-degree scalp burns are not our objective), but you do use comfortably warm water, not tepid. That same hot water that loosens the debris also stretches your hair somewhat, so you must always finish with a cold water rinse to help the hair contract and make the cuticle once again flat. Concentrate most of your energy on the new growth closest to the scalp, where most of the gunk collects. Since the ends are the driest (because they're the oldest part of your hair), they should be subject to less detergent action.

For Oily-looking Hair

If you need to shampoo every day, you're probably fighting odor, not soil. Oil at the scalp turns rancid, and rancidity produces a less than fresh smell. But since the middle and ends of your hair may be a bit faded and processed, you don't want to scrub with a vengeance daily. Unless you live in a highly polluted area, there just isn't that much dirt to be removed on a daily basis.

℞. *One sudsing is plenty* for every-morning shampoo fans.

For Dry Hair

Whether your hair is naturally dry, or drier, more brittle, and dull because of processing, you won't have to wash as frequently as the oilies to keep your hair looking and smelling clean.

℞. *Vary your shampoo regimen* (hair doesn't respond as well to the same shampoo after a while—it craves a change) as long as your chosen bottle is for cleaning dry-looking hair. Note: No matter how oily your hair usually looks, if you've had a perm, your processed hair now looks drier and must be treated accordingly.

For All Hair

℞. *No matter what type of hair you have,* if you have hard water, spend more time rinsing than you do cleansing or you'll leave behind a film that will keep your hair dull and dirty. One hard-water antidote is EDTA. Dr.

Albert Shansky, consulting cosmetic chemist, recommends you look for a shampoo containing this ingredient, which deactivates the scum-causing aluminum and magnesium present in hard water.

How to Dry

A brisk rub with a towel may bring a glow to your body, but it's too harsh for your hair. *Pat* hair dry with a towel, then wrap the towel around your head to collect excess moisture. Let it sit for 15 minutes, then blot hair with a second towel and set or continue with your electrical drying appliance if you have no time to let hair air-dry.

A Few Final Words about Shampoos

If your shampoo gets rid of everything, including most of the glow and sheen, it's actually doing its job. It takes Nature a day or two to replace the lost sebum that lubricates the scalp and hair and creates shine—which is why you may feel you can't do a thing with your hair right after you've washed it. You can't, because clean hair, especially if it was dry to begin with, becomes flyaway. Remember, shampoo is not a do-all product. It cleans, but to treat the hair, especially hair that no longer has the gleam of youth, you have to go further.

CREAM RINSE . . .

works to de-tangle hair after washing, controls static and flyaway hair, softens hair.

YOU NEED IT IF:

You find your thick hair difficult to de-tangle after shampooing and you seem to pull too much hair out in your attempt to get a comb through.

Your hair is flyaway, especially in winter when static electricity is more of a problem.

After washing, your hair becomes unmanageable and won't take a set or take to blow drying.

(*Special feature:* Cream rinses are acid-balanced to help close the cuticles opened by detergent shampoo.)

STAY AWAY IF:

You have limp, fine hair. The last thing you need is the softening produced by a cream rinse.

Exception: If you have limp hair that nonetheless snarls, you can get the de-tangling effect without undue softening by using a *concentrated* rinse that you *dilute* with water. Try diluting it twice as much as the manufacturer suggests—if it still de-tangles, you'll accomplish your goal with less "limp-producing" residue.

You have oily-looking hair. You don't need another coat of grease.

Your hair looks oily at the scalp, where new growth is coming in, but difficult to manage as the hair gets longer? Don't pour the cream rinse over your head, just use it on the middle and ends of your hair.

Your hair looks normal, except for frazzled ends near the top caused by frequent blow drying (my problem). When I use a cream rinse, my frizzies lie flat and behave, my hair looks sleek and unbroken. There is one drawback: I wash my hair every other day, and on the second day it does look a bit oilier than it otherwise would, but for me it's worth the trade-off.

CONDITIONER . . .

Hydrolized animal protein is the most important ingredient. It coats the hair shaft, helping to heal and close defective cuticles temporarily, thus promoting shine; conditioners also temporarily help split ends look less so by filling in the damaged, burst cuticle (I told you the cuticle was the key!) the length of the hair shaft, giving strength to hair that's been seriously weakened. Oils in the formula help fight the dry, brittle look, and acid helps close the cuticle the protein is filling in.

YOU NEED IT IF:

Your hair is dry-looking because your scalp does not provide as much oil as it used to.

You've overpermed, carelessly colored, overheated, and undertreated your hair.

Your hair is fine or thinning. Conditioners that contain protein coat the shaft and add a bit of thickness to each hair's width.

Note: Many conditioners also contain balsam, which is not a protein (it comes from a tree) but is an oil that effectively sticks to or coats the hair, adding a bit of bulk.

STAY AWAY IF:

Your hair is damaged but oily-looking. Keep the conditioner *away* from the hair nearest scalp: condition from mid-shaft to ends only. You must also cut back on heat appliances and processing, unlock trapped scalp oils with massage, then brush gently but thoroughly so your own oil will work its way from the scalp down to the ends.

Further Conditioning Cues

Read the label so you can match the cause with the proper conditioning cure. There are conditioners geared to help overcolored and overpermed hair. There are also products formulated to fight heat damage; these you apply before you use your curling iron/blow dryer.

A word about using: Treatment products, unless otherwise indicated, are not meant to be applied to the *scalp*. It's your hair they're treating and coating. So start at the ends, where the damage is greatest (where the least virginal of hair hangs), and work your way up as far as necessary. If your perm is growing out, for example, that 2 inches of new straight hair protruding from the scalp can be left alone. Instead, concentrate the conditioner on the hair that's drier-looking; applied any other place, it will be useless.

A 60-second instant conditioner, the kind you rinse right out, can be used regularly to give your hair more strength and elasticity. If your hair is dry-looking, dull, or damaged, use it more often than if your hair just needs a little boost.

The conditioning packs that you leave on 15 to 30 minutes contain additional emulsified oils that can be absorbed by hair that has become brittle, overdry, and "crisp"-looking. But if you use these deep-conditioning products too often, your hair will just get super-dull as well as heavy-looking and -feeling—you have to use your common sense (and look at your hair) to know when you're doing too much of a good thing.

A note for long-hairs: Even if your hair is healthy, the ends have been subjected to environmental excesses, heat, and mechanical abuse. Condition the bottom third of your hair as a preventive measure.

How often should you condition your hair—and with what? Only you and your hairdresser will know for sure because you have to tailor a conditioning program to your own very *individual* hair needs. Your regimen might run from never to twice-a-week instants (important if you have a perm or tinted hair) to a monthly deep-conditioning treatment (crucial if your hair looks like horse fodder) to a twice-monthly pack (if your tresses look as if they belong to someone old enough to cackle) to any combination of the above.

But how do you know if your efforts are paying off?

By comparing your hair before and after conditioning. Take a ½-inch section of de-tangled preshampooed hair between your thumb and forefinger. Run your finger along the entire length of the hair. Does it feel rough, dry? If so, the cuticle is probably raised. Now, after you've shampooed, conditioned, and combed hair, take another ½-inch strand. Does it glide easily through your fingers? Does hair still have some bounce, or is the conditioner so heavy your hair feels weighted and draggy? When your hair is dried, does it look shiny—or greasy? The more thoroughly you examine the hair, the better your chances of using a conditioner that will work for you.

THICKENERS: A "SPECIAL CASE" CATEGORY

Thickeners don't help condition your hair, but they do help camouflage thinning or fine hair by creating the illusion of added volume. If your hair is born-thin or thinning and you feel your body-adding protein-based conditioner is not effective enough, this newest of hair-care products will help. How? By coating your hair with bulk-adding resins and polymers like PVP (originally used as a plasma substitute during World War II), which will add still more width to individual hair shafts and make the space between hairs look less noticeable. Thickeners remain in your hair between shampoos.

CHAPTER 11

❦❦❦

From Past-Its-Prime to Prime-Time:
How to Style Yourself
a 10-Years-Younger Head of Hair

The preamble to fantastic, young-looking hair is getting it in the best condition you can, but a head of healthy hair isn't the end. It's just the beginning of a process that includes cutting, setting, coloring, perming—whatever finishing steps you must take to make your hair look terrific.

Why all this attention to hair? First, because it's the easiest part of your total packaging to change. Second, because your hair is one of the first things people notice about you. It frames your face, and if the "picture" itself is showing a little wear and tear, any art dealer will tell you that an attractive frame can give a more expensive look to the most ordinary painting.

But you have to treat your hair differently now and be prepared to invest a *little* more time (note: I didn't say hours) to rejuvenate what you've got. If you're still getting by with a daily shampoo and a quick blow dry, you may soon notice your hair no longer responds to this mini-regimen the way it used to.

You say you are zealous about care and conditioning, yet your hair still hasn't bounced back to its state of youthful innocence? Not to worry. The correct styling elements can give your hair (and your face) a really incredible lift.

What should you do with your hair? The following information, culled from my seminar notebooks, should cover just the topics you want discussed.

HAIR AS CAMOUFLAGE

I've been wearing my healthy, thick hair brushed back to show off my interesting hairline (my widow's peak is all I have in common with Liz Taylor). But lately all I notice are slight crow's-feet and suddenly appearing lines. I feel like I need a change. Suggestions?

You can *take comfort* in the fact that no one else studies your face as microscopically as you do, and you can *take charge* of the situation by learning to use your hair as *camouflage.* The right hairstyle can effectively lead the eye away from those incipient over-25 changes that appear almost unnoticeably on our faces. Up until this book was written, most authorities dealt almost entirely with the relationship between hairstyle and face shape. But for you, that kind of information is no longer enough. As the years past 21 start to pile up, you can (and should) style your hair to hide and de-emphasize first signs of aging.

Remember, a good cut and styling should make *you* look younger and better—not just your hair. Consider the following trick-the-eye prescriptions:

℞ *to soften forehead lines.* Wear bangs. I haven't seen my forehead for years! Whether curly, curved, or straight, full bangs effectively hide obvious lines and furrows. If you have just a few expression lines, strategically placed wisps, pulled down onto your forehead, may be all you need. Bangs are too

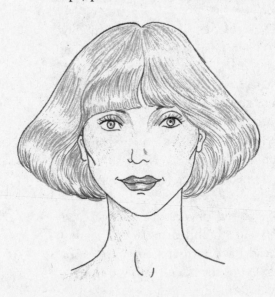

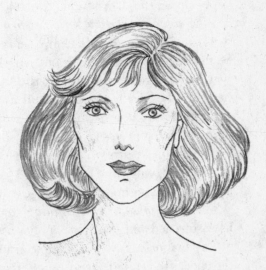

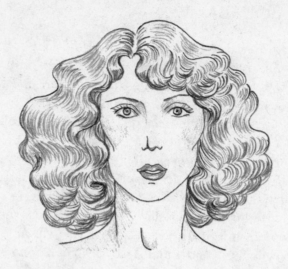

severe for you? The curls provided by a soft perm can be coaxed over your forehead. Hair pulled forward can also disguise a slightly receding hairline.

To style full bangs, try this hairdresser trick. First, brush bangs back off your forehead with the rest of your hair, blow drying as you go. Then brush bangs forward and blow dry them from above. The result: a sleek close-to-the-forehead look. For a soft curve, hook your round styling brush through bangs and aim your blow dryer at the brush.

℞ *to soften and camouflage crow's-feet.* Have your hair cut in dips, waves that fall naturally over the sides of your face—while you're framing your face, you'll also be covering some of that crow's-feet crinkling. A "surf" or "bowl" haircut with long bangs can hide some eyelid wrinkling, as well as problems on the sides of your face (just make sure you can still *see!*).

℞ *to camouflage a less than firm jawline.* If you have the beginnings of jowls and a slight double chin, you're exercising to help them along, but let's be realistic enough to check out what camouflage can do. Consider soft casual waves or a pageboy to cover up the jaw-meets-neck region, and aim for a little height at the crown, to lead the eye away from the problem.

Build height into the crown with your blow dryer. When hair is 90 percent dry, aim your head to the floor and brush and dry all hair against the direction of growth. Now, flip your head back into an upright position and finish drying on a lower "style" setting. Note the added volume up top, accomplished without hair damage or very dated teasing.

℞ *to camouflage a pudding-round face.* If your whole face seems to have softened and your cheekbones have disappeared as well, study the make-up lessons in Part Six. In the meantime, try bringing your hair forward on the cheeks to camouflage softening features.

Take It from Terry

Do you want graphic illustrations showing exactly how a change of hair can give you 10-years-younger style and pizzazz while camouflaging first signs of aging? Study the color photos following page 194 and notice the way the right style can give any woman a younger, more pulled-together look. The women pictured are far from old, but the wrong style ages them. Read the accompanying how-to commentary offered by scissor wizard Terry Foster, who provides an in-depth study of the whole hair-as-camouflage concept.

Terry is a famous and talented New York hair designer and consultant who specializes in creating image changes for film, TV, and magazine bookings. Since you may be considering changing your own life role, it's important for you to understand to what (great) extent a new hair look can contribute to your new image.

Terry says, "Hair is the last thing about herself a woman changes." Hopefully, you'll decide it's one of the first things about yourself you'll want to transform.

Of course, camouflage isn't the only consideration. Your hair can make you look older if you hang on to a hairstyle that no longer works for you, or you adopt the belief that once you turn 30, it's time to chop off your hair (not to mention your head). Consider the following admittedly personal rules:

□ Avoid the severe blunt cut, the chin-length "helmet." Short, geometric styles work best with young faces. Otherwise, they can make you look tough and battle-hardened.

□ I'm all for permanents, but leave tight little screw curls to Little Orphan Annie. Softer curls look far better on elegant women.

□ Don't pull your hair straight back in a bun without considering the consequences. To complement slicked-back hair, you must wear a complete, dramatic make-up, have or know how to create high cheekbones, possess smooth skin and the regal carriage of a *Vogue* model. Otherwise you will be drawing unwanted attention to every little facial line and you may end up looking like a headmistress in a 19th-century boarding school. Frankly, that's one dream I've never had! When you're 30ish, a little hair framing your face makes you look younger.

□ Don't wear very "done" hairstyles—unless you want to look done in. Literally uptight hairstyles—twisted, wrapped, and overly designed —all contribute to a formal, matronly look. Ditto for hair that doesn't *move*, so don't overuse hair spray.

- Don't wear "cute" barrettes and bows in your hair—unless you want people to think you're in your second childhood.

- Don't color your hair like a crazy person! Wild shades will make you look like a demented *Sesame Street* character. If you choose *I Love Lucy* red, "Dagwood and Blondie" blond, "Pocahontas" black, or "Thunderbird Wine" purple, you will definitely look more bizarre than beautiful.

- Teasing is aging. Period. If your hair is thin and you're teasing it to produce volume, you're wearing the wrong style.

- Adopt a look of *planned* carelessness. Anything that smacks of a highly styled coiffure that entails spending long hours under the dryer is aging. You should look as though you languorously stepped out of bed, ran a comb through your hair, and emerged with a swingy, lively hairstyle (would that it were so simple!).

- Finally—and most important—*don't automatically abandon long hair*. Any woman can wear long hair at any age if it is becoming and she has the hair for it. For myself, I find long hair more and more essential for maintaining a young look, especially as the rest of me starts to fray a bit around the edges. But it must look right, and not be *too* long, or it will make you look silly. Shoulder-length or a little beyond is not beyond reason, but I no longer picture myself scampering into the sea, a hibiscus blossom behind my ear, hair trailing past my waist.

　　You have to care for long hair differently now than you did when you were a young girl, but it's worth the effort, because short of an exquisite face and flawless body (both rather difficult to come by), there's nothing sexier or younger-looking than a mane of shoulder-length hair.

PRESCRIPTIONS RE THE CARE AND CODDLING OF LONG HAIR

℞. *If your hair has thinned with time*, or if you've never had thick hair, cut it. The weight of long hair will make thin hair appear even thinner around the scalp. Remember, a mane of long, full hair is sexy; mangy, stringy long hair is awful.

℞. *Use the correct cream rinse* and use it correctly. Just putting a comb through long hair can be a tress-traumatizing experience, because the cuticle, especially near the end, is old and brittle. To avoid the snarling and static that makes combing difficult, you'll need a cream rinse. But if you find your rinse leaves your hair too limp, use an extra-body shampoo first, then dilute your cream rinse with water and work it through hair from the middle of the strand down to the ends. This way, the hair nearest the crown, where you need body and lift, won't be oversoftened.

℞. *Take care of split ends.* Long hair is most prone to "splits," because it's more difficult to handle when blown dry, and the ends have been exposed to heat, environmental pollutants, the vagaries of weather, coloring, and other processes for weeks. Of course, the right wash and care regimen will do a great deal toward preventing the splits, but a haircut every six weeks or so is essential to build in shape and style and get rid of the ends that can't be salvaged. Besides, long hair that is left to get scraggly looks much worse combined with a postgraduate face than it does on a cherubic, unlined 20-year-old.

℞. *Use a wide-toothed comb* if you want those long hairs to stay attached to your head. Fine-toothed combs pull out too much hair while they're de-tangling. Your comb should be tortoiseshell (you shouldn't have to pay more than five dollars or so for the tortoiseshell used by hair-conscious models: Speert, Inc.'s No. 15 is a favorite stocked in drugstores). In any case, avoid sharp teeth and metal. The movement of metal against your hair encourages static electricity; pointy teeth encourage breakage.

℞. *Don't overbrush your hair;* do use a natural bristle brush.

℞. *Cut your use of blow dryers, curling irons, and electric rollers in half.* The last thing your no-longer-young long hair needs is a daily attack by the heat brigade. If a smooth look is your goal, adopt the practice of head wrapping. Set the hair at the crown on one or two jumbo rollers. Wrap the rest of your damp hair around your head, clipping in place as you go. You're actually using your head as a giant roller. When hair dries, unwrap (leaving rollers in place), dampen again slightly, and rewrap in the other direction. When dry, unwrap, remove rollers, and brush for a sleek style.

If you like the look of cascades of waves and your hair is in good condition, it's not too late to aim for that "*Cosmopolitan* girl" look. But unlike the 23-year-old models, you want to minimize the need for using hand-held appliances after each wash. You can try making giant pincurls or using "juice can" rollers. In other words, you have to *set your hair.* That's right—rollers, clips, the whole deal. I'll talk about techniques as soon as I answer the following camouflage-related question.

CONSIDER PROPORTIONS

I love the look of short, curly hair but since I've put on a few pounds, my head no longer seems to fit with my body. . . .

You've hit on a key that even the most fashion-conscious women often ignore. Your head must be in proportion to the rest of you, and as your body begins to change shape a bit, your hairstyle must compensate. Consider these prescriptions.

℞. *If you're now a bit wider* through the hips and thighs, you need a little more fullness at the top—around your hair—to balance your silhouette. Otherwise, you'll look like a pyramid, which is stunning only if your feet are anchored to the sands of the Sahara.

℞. *If you have broad shoulders*, wear your hair a little longer (at least 1½ inches below your ears) so you don't present a mannish appearance.

℞. *If you're elegantly elongated*—perfectly tall and slim—you can wear any sleek style. But too short and severe will make your face look too small and unimportant in proportion to your torso.

℞. *If you're short* (I prefer the word "petite," since I'm only 5 feet 3½ inches), the length of your hair isn't important, but the volume is. Too many curls and waves and too much height will be too overpowering. Whatever the length, opt for swing instead of lots of bouncy curls.

℞. *Wearing your hair back and up off your neck* will give you a sophisticated look and make you look a lot taller—but don't do it unless your neck is smooth, you have no hint of a double chin (check your chin in a side-view mirror), and you have good bones visible on your face. (These requirements rule out most of us!) And don't equate height with little curls piled high on top of your head—nothing is more 1950s.

℞. *If your bosom is becoming more prominent*, you'll look out of kilter with a short little "do," whether curly or straight. You need softness and volume in your hair to balance out the curves on your body.

GET SET

I've been wearing my straight hair in a chin-length blunt cut with a center part for quite a while—but my hair is thinning a bit; what's an alternative?

If your hair is getting a wee bit sparse, the first thing you have to do is eliminate your train-track part; a straight line focuses attention on the scalp showing through. Try a casual, tousled kind of look as opposed to all one length; the latter seems to drag hair down and make thin hair look even stringier. A good cut will be your base, with proper layering building in much of the swing and bounce.

But since you want to cut your use of hand-held tools in half, to get this look you must learn to *set your hair*. This is radical advice for those of us who went from the Pepsi Generation to the blow-dry generation, but unless you want to gaze in horror at a hairbrush laden with loads of locks every morning, you'll follow my simple, basic set technique once or twice a week. It will take just 15 minutes to complete, and the results will last a few days. Hair that's been through years of wash-and-wear treatment (including fanatic conversion to the appliance revolution that's responsible for so much heat damage) needs a reprieve now and then.

But you have to set your hair differently today from the way you did when you were a girl. No more sleeping on your nose with a head full of brush rollers—hopefully you have more interesting things to do at night now.

Don't worry about complex setting instructions. The pattern that follows can be combed out into a variety of styles, and it's all you really need to know if you have short- to medium-length hair.

Equipment/Techniques

Start with a clean, damp head. Whether or not you need a setting lotion, be it the time-tested liquids and gels or newer blow-dryer types, depends on how your hair responds to its use. Setting lotion may be too much after conditioners, cream rinses, et cetera. You have to experiment.

The looseness and softness of your look depend on the size of the roller, how much hair you put on each, and how much time you leave the rollers in your hair. You want smooth, plastic rollers. Wire mesh or brush rollers are easier to set, but they're disastrous for your hair. You won't use teeny-tiny rollers anymore—they make tight little ringlets that are more aging than elegant. You have thinning or fine hair? Medium rollers should be as large as you can get. If you have normal hair, you can use larger rollers to create a soft, face-framing look.

Whether you have thick or thin hair, don't try to put too many hairs on one roller; you'll either be tugging hair away from its natural resting place (thereby inducing premature death) or wasting your time with a messy set, which will lead to a messy finished look.

If your roller dexterity is nil when you first begin, end papers will help keep all the hair in place.

The right type of pins is equally essential to maintaining hair health. Tortoiseshell bobby pins are kindest to your hair. If you use the metal variety, be sure the ends are coated; when that little ball of coating falls off, throw the pin away—or throw your hair away.

You may prefer using clips to make pincurls. These should be rubber or blunt-tipped, rustproof, and open in design so air can circulate through.

When you're ready to wind, start by holding the chosen strand firmly, at an angle straight out from your scalp. But don't wind the roller so tightly that you feel your hair lifting away from your head. Remember, you're setting your hair to prevent damage, not encourage it.

The Pattern

Section off the center of your head from crown all the way back to the nape (the chunk you'd have left if you were shaving off the rest à la the Mohicans). Start at the forehead line and roll all hair back and under—using three or four rollers at the crown, however many more are necessary to do the rest of the center back of the head. Next, do hair framing the sides of your face. Hair here is thinner, so rollers will be smaller. Continue rolling the rest of the back of your head in a downward direction. Set those wispy hairs at the nape of the neck in pincurls.

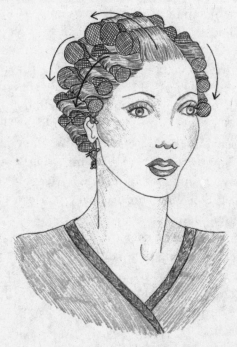

Whether your hair is fine, thinning, average, thick, you can follow the above pattern. If you are blessed with average or fuller hair, you can put in a straight part. With this versatile set you can wear your hair pulled forward, up, under, swept back—it all depends on how you style it as you brush.

Drying and Styling

Moisturize your face, then sit under a bonnet hair dryer set on medium-high heat. Since you are setting your hair damp, but not sopping wet, drying won't take that long. Turn the control to cool before turning the dryer off. Cool air will help you absorb the dampness produced by perspiration, so three extra minutes on cool before you remove the rollers will hold your set longer.

While using a hooded dryer is certainly not the best of all possible worlds for your hair, this necessary evil has certain advantages over the blow dryer.

Namely, heat is dispersed evenly over your whole head, not concentrated for too long in one spot as can happen with a "gun" dryer. Bonnet heat doesn't get as close to your scalp, so there's less chance of hairline breakage. Bonnet dryers usually provide more heat settings to choose from than the hand-held variety, so you can customize the heat flow to your individual needs.

After drying, unwind curlers and use your hairbrush gently to coax hair into a casual style that will give you the appearance of thicker, more voluminous locks.

℞. *For a firm set* that still produces soft waves, spray hair lightly after you remove the rollers, but *before* you brush your hair. This produces a soft look with body, whereas if you spray your hair *after* you've finished styling it, it will look too stiff and "coiffed."

The Perfect Pincurl

While cutting down on hand-held styling tools makes sense in theory, in practice I can't think of an alternate way to get those waves I like.

If your hair needs a boost to keep its curl in place, large pincurls may do the trick. Pull a damp strand of hair firmly (but gently) from the scalp, holding it as if you were about to put it on a roller. Instead, wind the curl around your finger. Slip the curled hair off your finger, pinning it flat against your head. Make sure the end of the strand is tucked into the curl before pinning. The smaller the curl, the tighter the wave; large pincurls give soft, smooth waves.

I use this appliance-substitute method when I'm working or vacationing in a humid or tropical climate. I make very large curls that take about 6 extra-large bobby pins to hold in place. The pins do leave "ridges" in the hair when it dries, but I consider this a styling plus: the ridges and crinkles give a very contemporary curly-wavy hairstyle. For sleeker waves, use extra-large smooth clips instead of bobby pins. One or two clips are enough to clamp even outsized curls.

HOW TO AVOID HEAT STROKE

Now that I've spent a good part of this chapter damning hand-held hair appliances, I want to confess that *I love them*. They've simplified my life greatly, and I would gladly give up my food processor before I'd give up my blow dryer.

But while my teen-age daughter uses her gun dryer daily and still has long, healthy, shiny hair (on her head—not on her brush), I have reached (and I suspect I'm not alone) that stage (or is it age?) when my mirror tells me my hair is no longer indestructible.

I've already said you must cut your use of these appliances in half (unless you want to make Baked Cuticles the hair-raising specialty of the house). If your hair is starting to lose some of its youthful exuberance, you have to weigh the convenience these tools provide against the condition in which they leave your hair.

Here, further thoughts on the use and abuse of the "big three"—dryer, curling irons, electric rollers. (There's no point in subjecting your hair to their heat on a daily basis.)

Blow Dryers

You don't need a blowtorch—a dryer that delivers 1000–1200 watts of power and soars to temperatures of 160°. When it comes to heat capability, less is more.

I've already suggested using a natural bristle brush for daily care. But if you use a brush when you blow dry, you'll also need a synthetic "vent brush"—air swirls through it, speeding the drying process.

Don't hold the dryer too close to your head—it has to stay at least 6 inches away from your hair.

Keep it moving—the longer it rests close to one section, the greater your chance of that clump of hair looking like overcooked spaghetti.

Always blow from the top down. If you blow from the ends up to the scalp, you'll be lifting the cuticle, causing split ends and frizzies.

Do use a conditioner specifically chosen to work with heat appliances—check the label.

Since hair must be 90 percent dry before you start styling, try to allow it to dry naturally as much as possible before you pick up the blower.

You need a lower speed to style than to dry, so turn down the control when most of the dampness is gone.

Electric Rollers

Buy a set that makes its own mist to minimize heat and "dry" damage.

Remove rollers carefully to prevent snarling.

If you want a hairset that lasts, realize that electric sets don't stay curled/waved as long as hair set conventionally.

Curling Irons

If the wand is too hot and you're not using it correctly, your hair can snap off in seconds . . . and I don't have to tell you how long it will take for hair to grow back.

Don't let it rest on your scalp. There must be a healthier way for you to indulge your masochistic tendencies.

Again, don't make the curling iron a daily ritual. All that heat pressed against the cuticles can crack them—leading to that dry, deadly, and dead-hair look.

Final thoughts: Don't choose a hairstyle dependent on electric rollers or irons for daily maintenance. These tools should be used only if your hair didn't come out right or you're in a hurry. Limit their use to twice a week *tops*.

THE TERRIFIC NO-SET ALTERNATIVE

Hair setting isn't for me; waves are. What will a permanent do for (and to) my hair?

If your dreams of soft, springy curls, cascading waves, and bouncy body have faded along with your hair color, "wavy hair" is one dream you can make come true without the services of your fairy godmother. (Like you, your fairy godmother may be starting to slow down a bit; she probably can't fly as energetically as she used to, so it's cruel to call the old dear out for every minor hair problem.)

Rather than waving a magic wand and singing *bibbity-bobbity-boo*, you can wave the rods and lotions that will give you a *permanent* new hairstyle.

Should you take the step?

A PERM IS FOR YOU IF:

You wear your hair pulled back because you can't figure out what else to do with it and your slicked-back hair is emphasizing lines and wrinkles.

You have bodiless hair that's dragging down your face, giving you a tired, older appearance.

You simply want a curly, wavy look, but you were born straight.

You have little time to fuss with your hair, but you want a definite style. A good perm means you hardly have to fool with your hair for months.

Your hair is healthy.

You have thin (fine) hair—the alkaline chemicals will raise your cuticle slightly, so each hair will look a bit fuller, giving you the look of added volume as well as style.

STAY AWAY IF:

Your hair is abused, overdamaged. (But if you get a good cut and embark on a serious conditioning program, you can turn yourself into a candidate.)

Your hair is thinning—if you have an *unusual* shedding problem, see a doctor, not a hairdresser.

You get bored with the same style. That perm will be visible for months, so if you like to go from straight to wavy to straight, plan on setting your hair for temporary waves.

You've decided you're a prime prospect, but you still have nightmares about the tears-provoking perm you had when you were 6 years old? Well, the process has vastly improved since then. But before I detail the benefits and drawbacks, let me outline how this better-hairstyling-through-chemistry procedure works.

I'll assume you're not interested in a learned dissertation on the structure of polypeptide chains and the function of disulfide bonds. In *nontechnical* terms, here's what happens:

Chemical changes. A perm is a two-step process using 1) waving lotion, and 2) neutralizer. The keratin your hair is made of contains four sets of bonds that give it shape. Three sets can be "broken" and reformed by wetting and setting.

The fourth pair, stubbornly strong bonds, are broken via the application of an alkaline cold waving lotion applied to your rolled-on-rods hair and allowed to do its bond-breaking work for a predetermined time.

Once the tough bonds that keep your hair straight are broken, a neutralizer is applied to the rods. This solution makes the bonds assume the shape of the rods—in other words, the bonds permanently re-form in the chosen curly/wavy pattern. The neutralizer is acidic, so it also helps counteract the effect of the alkaline waving lotion.

The time each of the two solutions is kept on your hair is crucial to the finished results. Timing determines how much curl you will have, how long the perm will last, and the state your hair will be in when the lotions are rinsed out.

Rod results. The style of your finished perm also depends on the size of the curling rods used. The larger the rod, the softer and looser the wave. Rod *placement* counts, too. Haphazard positioning yields haphazard results. But unlike careless roller placement, the unfortunate results won't wash right out.

Rod selection is also affected by the texture of your hair—smaller widths are better for fine to medium hair; medium and up rods work well on medium, coarse, and/or tinted hair.

Cuticle considerations. Porosity is yet another factor affecting permanent success. If your hair is very porous, it absorbs liquid quickly, because the cuticle is open, allowing fluids (i.e., waving lotions) to swim right in. Tinted, previously permed, or abused hair is porous, so it processes super-fast and must be tested as frequently as every minute to insure fantastic, rather than frazzled, results.

Your hair is still primly virginal, therefore you assume you've got one terrifically tight cuticle and nonporous hair? 'Tain't necessarily so! So the perm timing of even virginal hair must be monitored faithfully.

Or . . . what? How about a headful of frizzies or frazzled, spongy, matlike hair? All are distinct possibilities of overprocessing. Underprocessing is no picnic either. If you miscue the timing on the conservative side, your efforts will amount to nil, because your hair won't adequately curl.

If all of the above makes super-perming sound a bit more complex than the invention of microcomputer transistors, that's what I had in mind. I really think this process should be left to skilled salon professionals who perm dozens of heads a week, so they develop a sixth sense about timing, lotion strengths, rod size, et cetera. (Ask friends and strangers whose heads you admire where they had it done—everyone loves to have her hair complimented.)

Before you decide where to go, check the perms turned out by the best department store salons near you. Because of their size, they do perm after perm, and what you want is someone with lots of experience.

Of course, my pro-professional bias could be due to the fact that I am not known for my manual dexterity (besides, you can either have long acrylic nails or give yourself a perm; I admit—I chose the former!). Seriously, I do spend a great deal of time in salons, and I do see a great many clients who come in after the fact seeking aid for self-inflicted perm problems (it's easy to spot them; the women invariably wear a turban and a grim look).

If you simply have to do it yourself, and I don't encourage it, make sure you follow the at-home kit directions faithfully.

In the late 60s I wore my hair long and straight, but when I outgrew my flower-child stage, I also permed my hair. I love the new look, but my hair no longer shines the way it used to.

You've hit upon one unfortunate drawback of a curly perm: lack of shine. No, it's not entirely due to the chemicals (though they are somewhat anti-shine because the alkaline solution raises the cuticle, and you know you need a flat cuticle for sheen). The curls themselves are partly responsible. Since your hair is no longer straight, lying flat along the side of your head like a sheet, light no longer bounces off it with the same vigor.

The way you handle permed hair also contributes to lack of shine. You don't vigorously brush the curls from scalp to end, not if you want to keep the waves in place. Instead, you "pick" it out with an Afro comb (get one with plastic, not metal, prongs), which doesn't touch the scalp. One drawback of this no-brushing regimen: Sheen-promoting scalp oil doesn't get a chance to travel and coat the length of your hair.

How to Create Shine and Care for a Curly Perm

℞. *Substitute scalp massage* for the *verboten* vigorous brushing to conserve curl *and* get the natural oils moving.

℞. *Lather only once* with your shampoo, even if your pre-permed hair was oily.

℞. *Don't shampoo daily*. Ex-oilies, realize your processed hair has changed character. It's drier, so there's no longer that much grease to remove.

℞. *Use a protein-rich instant conditioner* designed for permed or tinted hair to help fill in your cracked cuticle, which in turn will add a bit more shine.

℞. *Don't put a comb or brush through a wet perm.* Towel dry excess moisture and let your hair dry naturally if you have the time.

℞. *No time? Dry your hair* the way they do in salons. Buy a 150-watt infrared light bulb. Ask your beauty salon where they get theirs, or look in the Yellow Pages under "Beauty Salon Equipment and Supplies." If there is such a beauty trade shop near you, pay a visit. While their main clientele are salon owners, the personnel are usually happy to fill consumer requests if you have something specific in mind.

℞. *Add shine* by rubbing a dab of Vaseline or Alberto VO5 through your finished hair.

Can I perm and color my hair?

Yes, if it's healthy. The perm comes first; wait 10 days before tinting. If your hair is already tinted, use a perm formula designed for colored hair. Since you are planning two treatments that will chemically change your hair, consult with a professional first, and at least let the salon do one process for your hair's sake (they really should do both). Exception: If you're also planning a double-process coloring job involving prebleaching, *change your plans.* Enough is enough! You don't want to submit your hair to too many alkaline processes.

Caveat: If you're having a perm, henna is out. It's a terrific coloring agent, but it mucks up the bonds involved in perming, and you don't want to muck up your hair.

CHAPTER 12

❦❦❦

First Gray and Other Sorrows: A Fail-Proof Hair Tint Selection System

If the advent of your seventeenth gray hair has depressed you more than any event since the breakup of the Beatles, your "friendly" divorce (you should have made him take the dog, who now bites any man who enters the bedroom), or the realization that the Robert Redford look-alike at work prefers the *male* mail clerk, you're obviously in a gray funk.

To rephrase Shakespeare (I might as well start at the top!), "To color or not to color—that is the question."

Rather than submit to melancholy and indecision, study the color compendium that follows, and you'll have all the information you need to decide and to do or have the job done exquisitely.

The Gray Funk Analysis

If experiences similar to the following have happened to you and you didn't smile bemusedly, you're ready to color your hair:

- When someone special introduces you as his "old lady," his friends treat you with the respect due his mother.
- You're in your early 30s, yet 21-year-olds offer to help you carry packages.

□ Though you're just 36, the younger girls at work ask you to help pick out Christmas gifts for their mothers.

□ Sharper than a serpent's tooth department: Your little girl says "Susie's mom looks much younger than you." (And you know that blonde is at *least* 10 years older.)

□ You're first-time pregnant at 33—and the only woman in your natural childbirth class who looks ready for menopause.

□ Your boss says "XYZ Cola" is a young account and though your ideas are marvelous, he's sending young Ms. Young to make the presentation.

□ The last man who engaged you in a harmless (though ego-boosting) office flirtation was old Mr. Carruthers—and he's color-blind.

□ They tell your husband he looks *fantastic*. Your compliment (if they notice you at all)? "I love the way the light picks up the silver in your hair."

I don't quite remember what triggered my personal hair color go-ahead decision; probably something as mundane as a long look in the mirror. I've been coloring my hair to add shine and drama (and, yes, cover first grays) for years—and I wouldn't do without it.

Hair signifies youth and sexuality. When you let your hair go, you're unconsciously saying "good-bye to all that," and even though you may be smoldering inside, you're giving off "I've given up" vibes.

I think only two kinds of women look terrific with gray hair: 1) The very young, who have prematurely grayed. In their case, the gray offers a dramatic, unexpected contrast to soft, unlined skin. 2) The over-50 women with good skin and thick, well-cared-for silver (rather than yellowed) hair.

But if you're an in-between woman following the usual helter-skelter graying pattern, I think you're doing yourself an injustice.

FIRST GRAYS

Women generally start to turn gray in their early 30s (with men, graying often isn't noticeable until the early 40s). The pigment-production process locked in each hair bulb slows down and stops, till the affected hair has no color—it's really white. How the white hairs look depends on the color they're reflecting off. If the rest of your hair is dark brown or black, the whites will look steel gray; if your hair is blonde or light brown, you'll look all-over mousy; redheads tend to develop a faded, rusty cast. In your mid-30s, in spite of these changes, you'll still be known as a blonde/brunette/

redhead—your hair isn't yet engulfed (the way it may become in your 40s) by gray, but it just doesn't look terrific anymore. Besides muddying up your natural color (which is already fading because of that three-letter word I'm tired of repeating), gray hair has no sheen—it's dull-looking.

Even if you have just a few grays, they tend to be more noticeable because gray hairs are often wiry and coarsely textured (even if the rest of your hair is not) so they stand out like candles on a birthday cake.

First graying usually begins around the temples, sides, and top of your head. It will look worse if it's scattershot through your hair than if it's part of a dramatic streak (the latter you may want to keep; the former—forget it!).

You should also know that blue-eyed, fair-skinned women can carry gray better than their olive-skinned, dark-eyed sisters.

But you needn't have witnessed the sprouting of even one gray to exercise your color option. If your hair has faded, you, too, may be ready for a change. Dull hair is not your imagination if: there are no highlights, even if your hair is healthy; conditioners don't replace the shine; color doesn't come back in the winter (so you can't blame the fading on temporary sun abuse).

COLOR YOURSELF YOUNG

If a look in your own mirror (not to mention your soul) has convinced you to give color a try, *color choice* is the first decision you must make.

If you're not sure where to begin, remember, the possibilities are *not* endless. You must cue the color to your genetic code, which means eye and skin color must be considered. If you stray too far, the results will look garish. *Example:* You have deep brown eyes and hair and olive skin? You'll look unnatural as a light blonde. Besides, the old-fashioned "bottle blonde" look favored by Roaring 20s film stars is as dated as bow lips and Betty Boop eyelashes.

It looks as though my Latin background dooms me from finding out firsthand if blondes have more fun. But I do want to cover my first grays and spark up my dark hair. What do you suggest?

What color will help you shed years and get a vibrant glow on?

In my attempt to sleuth out a fail-proof tint selection system, I cross-examined many experts from top salon hair colorists and dermatologists to my own make-up artists (they're very tuned in to color and its effect on women), and I found that their advice, coupled with my own years of self-experimentation and woman watching, jibed most closely with the tint research undertaken by the experts at L'Oréal, who suggest that every coloring candidate study her eye color and skin tones for first clues.

IF YOUR EYES ARE	CONSIDER
dark, reddish brown	red and copper blonde hair; medium copper hair; dark auburn hair
light, warm reddish brown	dark auburn hair; bronzed auburn hair; light, pearly pastels (without yellow)
blue	quite light; all medium and dark shades; silvery, pearly
gray-blue or hazel	ash-blonde, slightly golden (a bit of yellow)
blue-green with green predominating	red-blonde (without too much red)
yellow, golden	very light, warm gold hair

Marion Walsh, L'Oréal's technical education director, says that very dark shades accentuate the lines on your face; in general, it's better to opt for lighter tints when grays (which usually appear around the face first) come forth. Our skins either start to lighten or turn a bit sallow in our late 20s++, and lighter shades work better with both of these complexion changes.

IF YOU ARE STARTING TO GRAY, AND YOUR COMPLEXION IS	CONSIDER
fair	blonde or auburn shades; if hair is more than ⅓ gray, a soft ash-blonde will be more flattering
ruddy	ash-blonde or brown shades; if hair is graying go for soft ash-brown, and avoid any shades containing red
olive	deep auburn or mahogany shades; graying hair looks attractive with light brown; avoid any completely light, bright shades
sallow	coppery red or auburn shades give a glow to the skin; if hair is more than ⅓ gray, a beigy blonde shade flatters and dark shades should be avoided
neutral	golden blonde or coppery brown shades; if hair is starting to gray, a light brown shade is recommended

If you're convinced nothing but blonde hair will do (as I am for many women), pick your particular shade with care.

COMPLEXION	SHADE
fair	soft ash-blonde
rosy	deeper toasty ash
olive	medium to deep beige (are you sure?)
sallow	warmer beige
neutral	light blond or light golden

Finally, consider your natural hair color—the way it is now. Cut off a snip of clean, dry hair from underneath, at the nape of the neck (where it's most protected from environmental changes). You also have to study the hair in front, nearest your scalp (this hair you'll examine *in situ*—don't cut it off). You must examine both hair locations, because hair in front is usually one or two shades lighter than the rest of your head.

Make your comparisons by a north-facing window, which is considered true light (artists always set up their easels facing north).

℞ *for born blondes.* Stay within the light range (dark hair will offer too harsh a contrast with your fair skin unless you are very young), but don't go too platinum. You see few natural platinum blondes over the age of 12—platinums turn to honey—it's Nature's way of putting hair color in harmony with changing skin tones and (later) first wrinkles. Tone-on-tone blonde streaking (more about this later) is a dramatic way both to highlight your natural color and to conceal first grays.

℞ *for natural redheads.* You can run the gamut from fire-engine to deep auburn . . . but is fire-engine still for you, and why does natural bright red fade so soon? It fades to go with your changing skin. The translucent skin most redheads possess is thin, and thin skins start drying and lining early. Nature knows harsh or bright colors don't go with lines, so she speeds up your hair-fading process. When you start to fade or gray, you want to jazz up the gift you've been given with darker auburn highlights, not try to return to the burning-bush color of yesteryear.

℞ *for medium to dark brown hair.* Start your experimenting by going a shade or two lighter than the color nearest your scalp at the hairline—a bit of lightening will enhance your changing skin tone. Or you can match your own shade both to cover the gray and to highlight what you've got. But *don't* go raven-haired.

℞ *if you started life as a true brunette,* but now see your naturally black hair has faded a bit (not to mention the fact that it's flecked here and there with a wiry gray hair or three). Bring it back to your ultra-deep natural shade if your skin is truly unlined. But if you're starting to crinkle a bit around the eyes, Nature is telling you jet-black won't do anymore. You'd be better off to warm up your black hair with rich chestnut brown or deep auburn highlights that will cover the grays and impart a flattering glow to both your hair and face.

Listen to Terry and Leland

Before you decide "this is *definitely* the color for me," turn to the color insert, and study the "Time Machine" photos and the explanation in Part Six, Chapter 21. As you'll notice, at certain ages certain shades within a color range can be more flattering than others. As mentioned, proclaiming you want to be a redhead, for example, is not enough. You have to be more specific. Would you look best in a light auburn, deep copper, reddish blonde, or claret shade? Can you still be a true red-red, or will you look as though you're wearing a fright wig?

Since I want this chapter to provide you with as fail-safe a tint selection system as possible (within reason—you and your hair colorist must make the final analysis), I've shown in living (if not breathing) color the shade range that works best for the same women *at different ages*. It's no secret that the blatant blonde you can get away with at age 21 may differ from the blonde you should be when you tilt toward 40.

So if you want to trade your fading, do-nothing, or graying hair for a 10-years-younger color, study the photos and heed the advice offered by image changer Terry Foster and super colorist Leland Hirsch.

COLOR, TIME, AND MONEY

OK. I've picked my color, now how about techniques?

Before you hit the bottle, there are several additional points to keep in mind, and they all deal with how much effort (time and money) you're willing to devote to keeping your new color terrific-looking.

Hair may be dead, but it certainly grows. And you'll become very aware of the speed of the new growth as soon as you color your hair. Two-toned heads can be dazzling if you're talking about streaking, but there's nothing more unattractive than an inch of dark roots contrasting with the rest of your copper mane. If you have very dark brown/black hair and go blond, you'll need a retouch every two weeks. If you have light brown or quite gray hair, you may be able to get away with a retouch once a month (though every three weeks would be better).

So before you make any color change, you must be sure you have the time and patience required. If you have your hair professionally colored, you have to figure the price of the original job, plus the cost of frequent touchups.

Is it possible to get around the retouch commitment? Here, a few tips for prolonging the life of your color:

℞. *Change your hairstyle.* If you're wearing a look with a definite part, you can be sure the roots at the part line will offer a too obvious point of demarcation. With a part-free tousled, casual style the new growth is more hidden, and you may be able to wait up to a week longer between touchups.

℞. *Invest in inexpensive touchup tools.* Hair color sticks or crayons can be purchased wherever home coloring kits are sold; you just pencil over the offending roots. Soft eyebrow pencils that match your chosen shade can also conceal regrowth. If you have just a few grays, you might want to substitute these tools for a whole-head color job.

℞. *Stock up on temporary rinses.* Actually, these are downright *ephemeral:* The result disappears with your next shampoo. Still, they're useful if your new coloring is starting to fade or brassiness is showing up in your blonded hair, yet it's too soon for a retouch. Warning: If the weatherman predicts hurricane Bruce is just around the corner, remember, a pouring rain as well as a shampoo can wash these rinses right out of your hair (and right onto your clothes—many a beautiful dress has been stained by a sudden garden-party shower).

℞. *Substitute special effects* for whole-head processes. "Specials" include frosting, streaking, hair painting, sunbursting—the names are varied, but the processes are similar. Selected strands of hair are either pulled through a cap, sectioned off from the rest of your head by aluminum foil, or surface-painted. Once these strands are chosen, they are bleached, then tinted with a blonde toner, so your hair looks shot through with highlights. Since there is no one definite root line, *you can wait up to six months between treatments*, making specials a great time and money saver.

More on "Specials"

If you are light to medium brown haired, a faded blonde, or getting a wee bit gray, highlight/streaking can give you the look of blonde without the constant bother. Specials are also kinder to your hair, because although they are double-process jobs, only selected hairs are subject to alkaline chemicals, and the chemicals don't touch your scalp.

If more than one blonde toner is used, you can better duplicate naturally sun-kissed hair, because a close look at virgin hair reveals it may be the same *color* (i.e., brown), but it really encompasses several *shades* (perhaps from warm to deep brown to rust).

I think well-done special effects can effectively and efficiently help women drop 10 years. If you're ready to go ahead, go straight to a pro. True, there are at-home kits, but for all the reasons I've mentioned, you'll have great difficulty duplicating *chez vous* the dramatic results a trained colorist can coax from drab, washed-out, or first-grayed hair.

Exception: You have dark hair. *Skip this technique altogether*. The blonde toners will show up *white* in contrast to your dark hair, so you'll look as though your hair is ribboned with gray—not quite what the beauty expert ordered.

HOW TO RESHAPE YOUR FACE WITH HAIR STREAKING

When one beauty procedure performs *two* important functions, you know you're getting your time and money's worth. Such is the case with streaking; it not only gives you the knockout glamour blonding generates—it can also help reshape your face to camouflage structural flaws caused by time. If you have the hair color and skin coloring that will take to streaking, a canny colorist can help take care of the following (the difference in shading between the streaked and natural hair is exaggerated in the illustrations to give you a more exact streak placement guide):

Jowls and a double chin can be minimized by placing streaks along the crown and at the temples to draw the eye away from the lower third of the face.

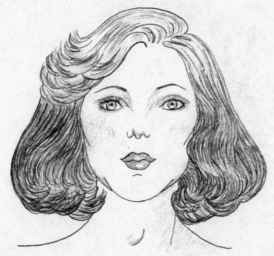

A drawn, hollow-cheeked face can be made fuller looking by concentrating streaks along the sides of your face and keeping hair swept back and upward.

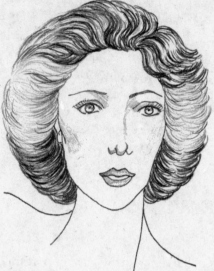

If you have tiny lines above the lips or deeper vertical "laugh lines" from your nose to mouth, streaks positioned lower on the face will distract the eye from these center-face problems.

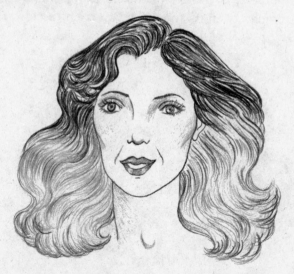

Streaking all around the face can help soften wrinkles and give a mellow glow to a complexion that time is turning sallow or dull.

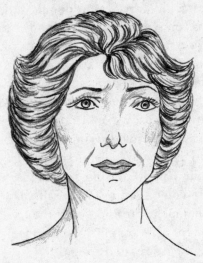

COLOR YOURSELF CORRECTLY

There are so many different types of coloring products available—how do I know which is for me?

To give you a clearer picture of what that profusion of boxes and bottles promises (and accomplishes), let me give you a quick techniques glossary.

I've already described the limitations of *temporary rinses*.

Semipermanent Processing

With "semis," the results last from four to six shampoos. When their life is over, they just fade gradually away, so you don't need to retouch roots. Semiperms contain no peroxide, so they're not hard on the hair. But no peroxide means no bleaching, so you can't lighten your hair; neither can you stray far from your natural color. What you can do is add some highlights to your own color, or cover first grays without altering the rest of your hair. If you're a mere babe in the color market and want to change *yourself*, start your at-home experimenting using "semi" formulas.

Permanent Color Procedures

There are two types, single-process and double-process blonding. With both, hair so tinted remains colored until you cut it off.

Type #1: Single Process. Hair industry stats say that 60 percent of the women who color their own hair do it permanently (the figure is probably higher in the salon), using a single-process technique. (I owe my gray-free aubergine hair to this process and my colorist. My own hair is, or was, a very dark, though faded, brown.) In one step, hair is both lightened (bleached) and colored, because peroxide is mixed with the tint base.

Single processing can take you several shades deeper or lighter than your natural color. If your hair is starting to show gray, hopefully you'll want to go a bit lighter. If you're getting more salt than pepper in the front but the grays haven't done much spreading over the back of your head, you may have to use two different tints for proper coverage—hopefully you'll let a skilled colorist do such complex camouflaging.

One-steps can also effectively color gray without changing your natural dark color—just choose a shade closely matching your original. You can even go from medium dark to medium blonde, but not from dark to pale.

Retouching involves parting and sectioning your hair (which isn't easy), and care must be taken not to color over previously tinted hair.

Single-process bonus: The slight alkalinity raises the cuticle, so if you have fine, thin hair your hair will actually look fuller, if you care for it properly.

Type #2: Double Process. You're determined to make a dramatic change from very dark to very blonde hair? You'll need the permanent technique known as double-process blonding. First, your hair must be pre-lightened, or bleached, so the red tones are removed. Your hair not only whitens, it becomes more porous, so it will be better able to "accept" the blonde toner in the shade you choose.

True, you may become a glorious golden girl, but your hair may also become very dry, brittle, and breakable, so you must care for it properly to keep it looking as soft and healthy as possible.

If your hair is mousy brown or quite gray, double-processing won't be quite as devastating to the hair shaft, because you won't have to submit to prebleaching for as long a period as the darker-haired.

SHOULD YOU . . . OR SHOULD THEY?

This is really a more crucial question than *Does she . . . or doesn't she?* As you've probably guessed, I think *they,* the salon professionals, should do permanent coloring if your budget will allow it (if not, ask a trusted friend for help; you really do need more than two hands). I have three reasons for giving the salon my vote:

Reason #1. Customized results. A good colorist can expertly blend several different tints to give you a natural-looking head of hair.

Reason #2: Covering gray. You'd think your gray hair would be *grateful* for a chance at new color. Instead, some grays are stubbornly resistant. The salon specialist can juggle techniques and timing to make sure your hair is gray-proofed when the job is finished.

Reason #3. Choosing the right shade. It takes experience to develop a trained color eye. A good colorist should be able to help you decide on just the hue (or hues) that will give you the results you want.

How to Choose a "They"

How do you know if you're placing your head in the hands of a true *artiste*, a coloring superstar? Watch the heads that are turned out by your favorite salon; ask women whose hair you admire, "Whodunit?" If you're planning to try a new salon for color, invest in a preview appointment for a less-expensive service (a wash and blow dry, perhaps), so you can unobtrusively study how their colorist (and the staff in general) operates.

Check the national beauty and fashion magazines or the women's pages of your local newspaper to see which colorists from your area are publicized. You only live once, and it's worth the investment it takes to get rich-girl hair color from a state-of-the-art professional.

Going It Alone

If you have always been good with your hair, and have yet to find a Mr. André to whom you would entrust your tresses, I have just three cautionary words:

FOLLOW THE DIRECTIONS

All of them. To the letter. If you need only one tint (rather than the subtler mix of a few) to achieve happy results, and you're planning a single processing, you'll *probably* be in good hands.

But if you've never bleached your hair (which is what "peroxide prelightening" is) or haven't attempted a double-process job since you were 16, give serious consideration to seeing a coloring pro. Your hair is no longer young (even though the rest of you may be just 27), which means it's more porous, less elastic, and probably not all of the same texture (especially if you have some scattered gray wires poking through), all of which means expert *timing and techniques* are crucial to avoid damage—and give you terrific hair color.

But whether you do it or they do it, you'll be responsible for the routine care of your new color (and your changed hair).

The Care and Feeding of Tinted Hair

℞. *Before your hair is colored*, make sure your scalp is healthy (no bumps, scaliness, scratches), it's been at least a week since your perm, and your hair itself is in good shape: split ends cut off, rest of hair supple and well conditioned. Don't color if suffering from unusual fallout.

℞. *After your hair is tinted*, cover up in the sun to prevent further bleaching and drying out; comb through a conditioner or use a bathing cap before swimming in chlorinated water.

℞. *Use a color-fast shampoo.* The acidic pH will help neutralize the effects of the alkaline chemicals necessary for coloring.

℞. *Don't shampoo daily.* Your drier, oil-drained hair no longer needs it. If you're a compulsive shampooer, lather just once.

℞. *Use an instant protein conditioner* after each shampoo to help temporarily close and coddle your raised and fragile cuticle.

℞. *Give yourself* a hot oil treatment like L'Oréal's Oleocap or a deep-conditioning pack like Clairol's condition* once or twice a month if your usual regimen still leaves your hair brittle and dry.

VEGE-COLORING

I'm anti-alkaline anything. You haven't mentioned henna.

An oversight I'm about to correct. Henna, the natural vegetable product used for some 2,000 years in the Middle East, has no harmful side effects, except garish results if used improperly (but that's true of any coloring product).

When used according to directions, on nontinted, nonbleached, nonpermed hair, the results can be fantastic. Henna doesn't penetrate the hair, so it won't provide enough depth of coverage if your hair is more than 15 percent gray. But it *can* highlight, condition, deepen, and dramatize hair that's suffering from first grays and/or other sorrows (specifically, fading).

If you're doing it yourself, understand that the henna and water pack you glop on your head will be messy. Make sure the label reads *natural* (not compound).

One terrific henna plus: It fades away gradually, so there's no root work to look forward to.

Other henna thoughts:

- It now comes in black, brown, and neutral as well as red.
- Neutral leaves your own color as is, but gives you added body and shine (add one whole egg for even richer results).
- Reminder: Henna and permanents don't mix. The former interferes with the bonds that are curled to produce the latter.
- Follow the instructions for timing and application, but if you're feeling adventurous, you can customize the color.

Custom #1: Deepen black henna by substituting strong coffee for the required water.

Custom #2: Boil tea, remove the bag, let it cool, and use the liquid instead of plain water. Result: Increased red highlights in dark brown hair.

Custom #3: For slight blonding (though henna won't take you from dark to light), add lemon juice to light brown henna.

- Leave bright orange henna to the very young, or rock stars.
- If you're aiming for an unusual plum or deep brandy color, see a professional. Henna is tricky to use, and you never know quite what will happen until you're finished, so if you dare to be burgundy, at least let the colorist figure out how it should best be done.

HELP!

Who can I turn to when nobody seems to know how I can quickly correct the too-blonde coloring I overzealously inflicted upon myself?

For answers to individual coloring problems (or for sound advice before you buy your first at-home kit), it's comforting to know that the personnel at L'Oréal are sitting by their phones and mailboxes, waiting to hear from you—and willing to provide topnotch technical information. Keep this phone number and address handy:

L'Oréal of Paris Products
Consumer Affairs
530 Fifth Avenue
New York, N.Y. 10036
Telephone: (212) 840-3900

PART SIX

WHAT
A DIFFERENCE
A DAY MAKES

What a difference a day makes!

Morning

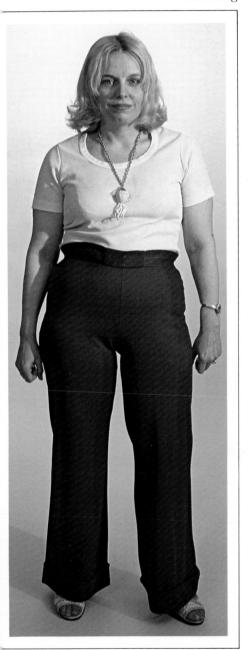

FROM SUPERMARKET
TO SUPERWOMAN

Same day, unretouched photo

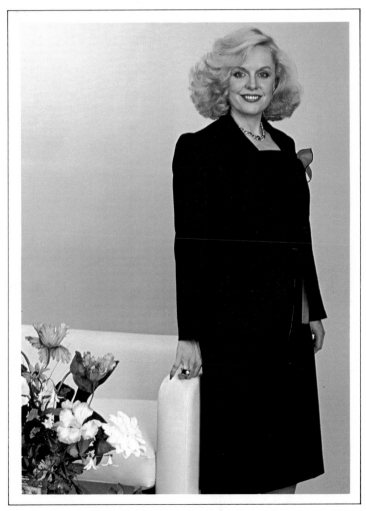

FOR FULL DESCRIPTION SEE PAGE 201

Morning

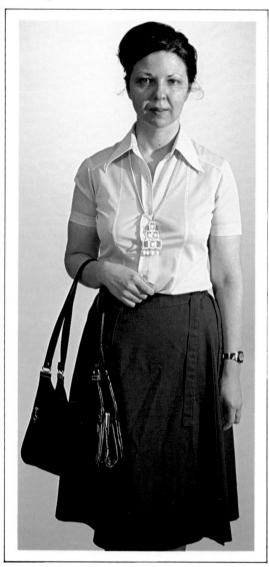

THE OVER-30
GLAMOUR GIRL

Same day, unretouched photo

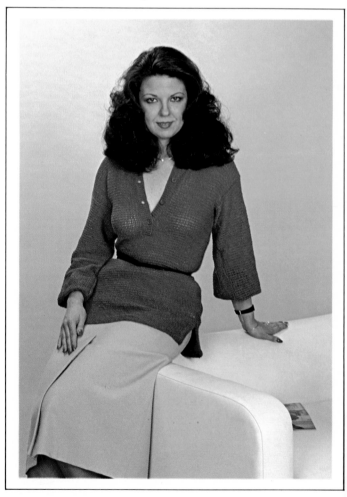

FOR FULL DESCRIPTION SEE PAGE 208

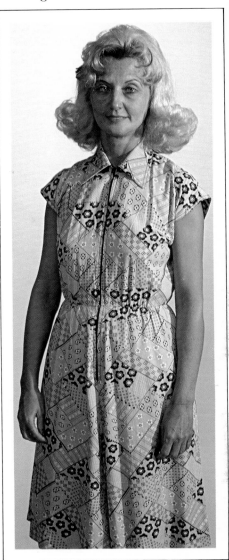

EARLY TO MID-40s
GRANDMA TO GREAT LOOKING

Same day, unretouched photo

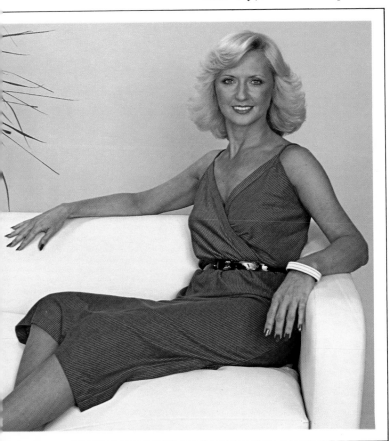

FOR FULL DESCRIPTION SEE PAGE 215

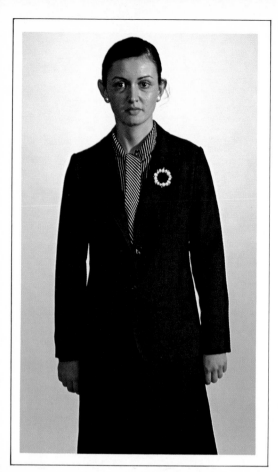

CAREER DRESSING:
MOCK MAN...OR DYNAMIC WOMAN

Morning

Same day, unretouched pho

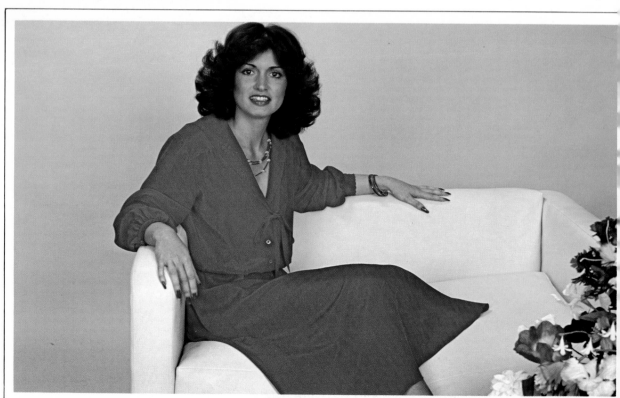

FOR FULL DESCRIPTION SEE PAGE 2

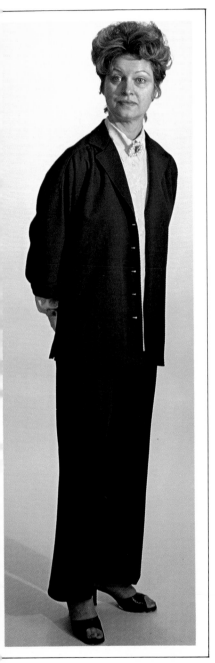
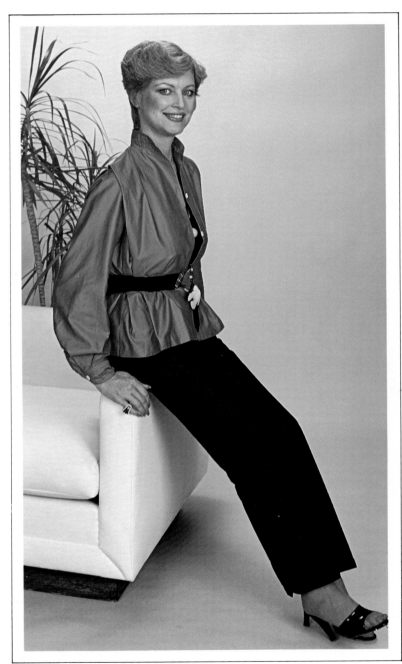

Morning   *Same day, unretouched photo*

FOR FULL DESCRIPTION SEE PAGE 238

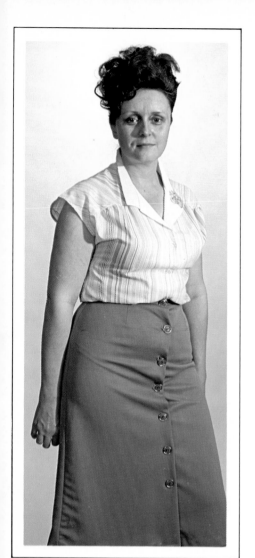

Morning

MOMMY, IS THAT YOU?

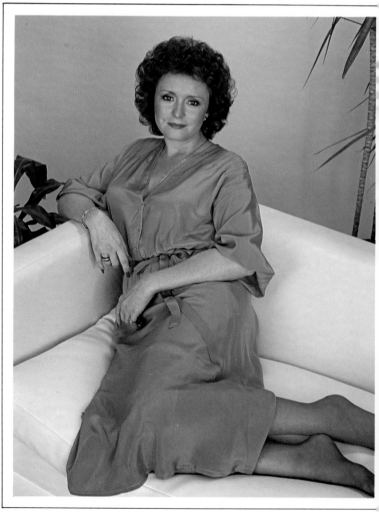

Same day, unretouched photo

FOR FULL DESCRIPTION SEE PAGE 244

OVER 55/
OVERSTATUSED/
OVERDONE

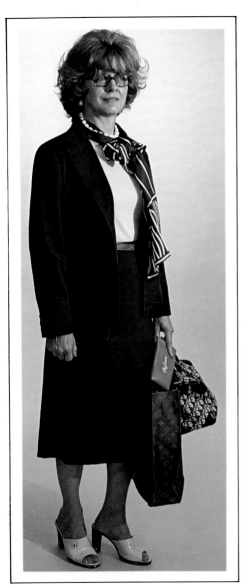

Morning

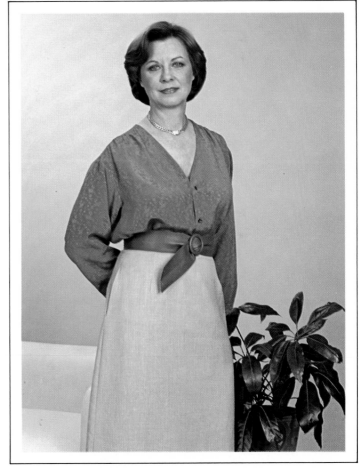

Same day, unretouched photo

FOR FULL DESCRIPTION SEE PAGE 252

THE HAIR COLOR TIME MACHINE:
HOW TO CHANGE YOUR HAIR COLOR AS TIME CHANGES YOU

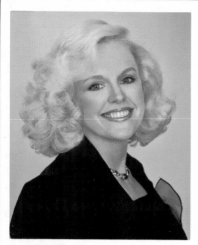

25-PLUS

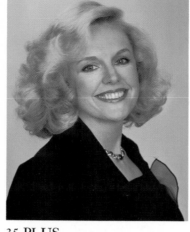

35-PLUS

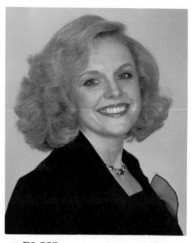

45-PLUS

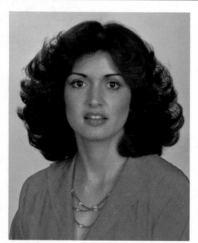

25-PLUS

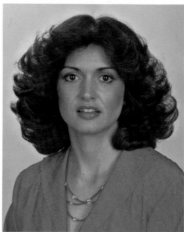

35-PLUS

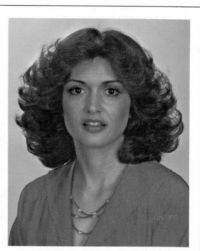

45-PLUS

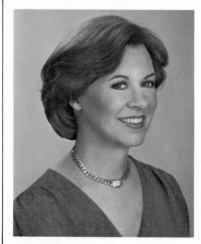

35-PLUS

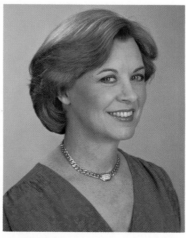

45-PLUS

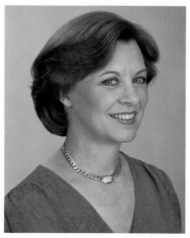

55-PLUS

CHAPTER 13

❦❦❦

The Making of
a 10-Years-Younger Image:
Immediate Same-Day Results

Are you a textbook case "split personality"? If you speak and think *young* but your appearance gives off other vibrations, your look is overpowering the woman you can be. When your mirror reflection is at odds with your desired self-image, you must adjust the outer you to match your young personality. It's actually an easier and more realistic goal to make yourself look years younger than to wait for old to be in!

No, you don't need to make a fifty-dollar-an-hour thrice-weekly appointment with your local therapist (no wonder psychiatrists can afford to have their ultrasuede couches re-covered twice a year) in order to make your inner and outer images unite. But you do need to learn the specifics that will allow your younger self to come out of the closet.

How long will this physical transformation take? I'm not talking about years of analysis (it's too late to blame mother—even if you are starting to look like her), months of strenuous exercises, and weeks of avoiding the fridge (though the latter two are important for long-lasting body changes). I am talking about the *immediate same-day results* you can achieve if you study, learn, and practice the art of *clever camouflage*. I know you can look years younger if you follow my "C.C." system, because I am in the business of creating new youthful images for women who want to change their lives —women who know that the best and easiest way for you to start improving your life is by changing your looks.

In politics, movies, TV, and big business, expert advisers and beauty professionals often are called in to repackage a person to fit whatever image he/she wants to project. In this chapter you will learn the same step-by-steps we teach these wealthy, powerful clients. You will learn how to update, improve, and camouflage every part of you to create an ageless package that can be marketed however you see fit—instantly.

THE HOW-TOS, ILLUSTRATED

Look and feel 10 years younger in one day . . . without plastic surgery, a two-hour tryst with Burt Reynolds, or a massive injection of Rumanian (or is it Bahamian?) sheep embryos?

If you're skeptical, study the A.M. and *unretouched* P.M. color photographs following page 194. I asked seven women from all parts of the country to demonstrate the common aging mistakes that rob too many women of young good looks.

The photos graphically support a truth I hold to be self-evident: *Each and every woman can be two women. Every woman has the option to look two ways.* In the morning photos, Option #1 is presented, with each woman portraying the good-looks errors made by many women who share a particular life style and "look style." I will detail for you the common hair, make-up, underwear, clothes, and accessory errors that add up to a catalogue of beauty and fashion faults that are *not* caused by time, but that do build up with time. Fortunately, these deadly flaws, *agers we do unto ourselves*, can be instantly undone, once you know how.

Option #2 will give you the know-how by showing you how the same woman can look when these errors are camouflaged, minimized, and (in some cases) completely erased. Whichever life style and look style you most closely identify with, you will learn how to make Option #2 a reality for yourself, because I will precisely define all the ways you can attack these drag-you-down problems in just one day. In fact, the solutions are so commonsense-simple to implement that once you learn them, you will be able to shed years as naturally as a lizard sheds its skin.

CATALOGUE OF ERRORS: THE SAME-DAY COUNTERATTACK

The self-inflicted errors are numerous, but so are the remedies. You will personally join the ranks of the in-between women who fight unnecessary age signs every day by learning how to:

- create the youth-keeping make-up and hair tricks I have gathered from my years in the beauty business (these tricks are successfully done every day in my world, so I know they will work in yours)
- de-emphasize and camouflage saddlebag cellulite bumps on the outside of your thighs
- handle heavy or loose upper arms
- make sagging breasts appear to stand at attention
- choose fabrics that tend to hold in less than firm flesh
- shrink a large waist
- use underwear, skirts, and dresses to narrow spreading hips and raise a slightly fallen derrière
- hide a spare tire and pot belly
- camouflage pendulous breasts and starting-to-sag neck
- cope with an overly ample body that time has softened and gravity shifted downward.

FLASH A GLAMOUR SIGNAL

Your problem is simply an allover lack of oomph, lack of style? The P.M. photos will show you how drama, style, and glamour can make you look younger. But understand that when I talk about glamour, I don't mean exchanging your everyday wardrobe for sequins, ostrich feathers, and rhinestones. I do mean developing a unique and personal fashion and beauty sense.

When you project a sense of good-looks glamour, no one will ask, "Is she 28, or past 35?" They'll just ask, "*Who is she?*"

I definitely believe that *style and flair* (my definition of glamour) are far more important than natural beauty, which is a gift from God. Of course, real born beauty is an obvious asset, but it will fade with time. That's why as you get older, it becomes more important to create an aura that time cannot dim. Great style and a look of your own are self-given gifts that you can create and keep forever.

If you understand how to give yourself the gift of glamour, you can alter your own good looks to your years, as one alters a garment to fit a changing figure. The photographs, as well as the illustrations and explanations in the following chapters, will give you the advice you need to give yourself this gift (it's really just a matter of avoiding certain obvious mistakes) *in one day.*

GLAMOUR: WHO'S GOT IT—HOW TO GET IT

At any social gathering you ever have attended, there usually is one "knock-out." She was probably wearing colorful, floaty and very glamorous clothes and dramatic, well-applied make-up; she had casual yet sexy, healthy-looking hair and good posture. But was she a classic beauty? You probably don't re-member if she had the bone structure and perfectly wide-set eyes of a true beauty, or if she was really very pretty, lovely, or just unusual looking. You don't quite remember—and it doesn't matter! You only remember that she was, in one way or another, great looking, because that's the image she presented—and that's the "package" you bought.

The *total package* is what you see and what you (and everyone else) remember. If Ms. Knockout is short-waisted and covers this flaw with a loose, flowing, no-waistline dress; if she hides a long waist with a fabulous two-inch vermeil belt from Morocco or keeps her less than slender waist cleverly hidden with a fashionable blouson effect—all you notice is the *final impact*, which was produced through careful attention to camouflage.

Clever camouflage is a kind of beauty brainwashing that should be adopted by every woman who is less than perfect; there are few who don't possess the prerequisite flaw or two necessary for membership in my Beauty Brainwashing Club. Once *you're* a card-carrying camouflagist, you'll be able to join those of us who know how to create what we haven't been given or are starting to lose: ageless good looks. The system that will give you the necessary knowledge is outlined below.

HOW TO USE THIS SUBTRACT-10-YEARS PERSONAL REPACKAGING SYSTEM

I hope I've convinced you that you can make a *quick* and startling difference in your looks if you learn how to use camouflage to re-create your own package and update your own image. To make it easy for you to assimilate all the seminar information I've gathered to explain these photographs, the first thing you must do is read through Part Six of this book in one sitting.

You will see that I have "repackaged" the women pictured with one goal in mind: to accentuate the positive, de-emphasize the negative, and cover up the boring in-between with a glamorous veneer. Remember as you read, all is fair in love, war, and camouflage, and all the world has to see is what you want it to see.

For each woman pictured, I've devised a five-step repackaging program, showing how all women who are willing to follow the same steps can develop a similar image. These steps are:

Step #1: The Strategy

In marketing a product (which is what you should consider yourself for image-changing purposes), agency people figure out just what the problems are that must be solved to make their client/product appeal to the target audience (in your case, the "target" may be a prospective employer, a mate who takes you for granted, or—most important—yourself). By studying the seven different featured strategies, you'll learn what to consider when planning your own self-marketing strategy.

Step #2: Hair Revitalization

A visual interpretation of the hair information presented in Part Five, with *specific* youth-adding changes that you and your hairdresser can and must make.

Step #3: The 29-and-Holding (Holding, Holding) Corrective Make-up Guide

Specific ℞s that will show you exactly how a cosmetic brush can be as effective as a plastic surgeon's scalpel when it comes to lopping off years. (Make-up is the ultimate camouflage. With it you can paint on a happy face, hide the ravages of time and tension, fill in wrinkles, or mask drooping.)

Step #4: Body Camouflage

The underwear, clothes, and color tricks that can instantly take you out of your problem body and immediately give you a younger, firmer look.

Step #5: A Little of the Young Razzle-Dazzle

What to look for and how to shop for the jewelry "musts" that will help you look like a young "status package."

BEAUTY BONUS:

THE HAIR COLOR TIME MACHINE—HOW TO CHANGE YOUR HAIR COLOR
AS TIME CHANGES YOU

Let's say you're a 35-year-old blonde who is still wearing the same hair-color shade you wore at 25. How should you update your hair color and make-up to enhance your changing skin? Or, maybe you're 25-years-old, "mousy brown," and toying with the idea of becoming a blonde. Is platinum for you? I have taken three of our women and shown how each one will look 10 years older and 10 years younger—complete with hair color and make-up, and a few wrinkles here and there. The result is a color analysis and fail-proof hair tint selection system for blondes, brunettes, and redheads . . . and I doubt if you've seen anything like it, anywhere. Study it, and you may be tempted to re-think your own entire make-up and hair-color palette.

To put yourself in the mood to get to work, have someone take a Polaroid of you the way you look right now—don't change your clothes, fix your hair or make-up. Unless you're that rare creature who wakes up with a song in her heart and gloss on her lips, you'll probably find some aspect of yourself that could use a little improvement.

Before you begin, I have one request: Bring no preconceived notions, fears, or hangups to your study of the following pages. In return, you will leave them with the knowledge that you can make yourself look 10 years younger and so much better . . . in one camouflage-and-beauty-packed day.

CHAPTER 14

⚜⚜⚜

From Supermarket
to Superwoman

Step #1: The Strategy

HIDE IT

In this morning picture, Rose strived to help me show you the "look" of so many women who let themselves go. This woman could be a busy suburban mother, a part-time worker–part-time homemaker with no time for herself. She could be the perennial optimist betting against all odds, admitting, yes, it did happen to my mother (heredity in body shape counts), but it could never happen to me. But "it" (the years and weight creeping up and settling in the most inappropriate spots) does happen to many of us. Although a diet is advised, camouflage is more important here. The results of hiding what you'd rather not show and accentuating good points are dramatically obvious in the afternoon picture. Here's our strategy in repackaging Rose to look 10 pounds slimmer and 10 years younger in just one day.

Step #2: Hair Revitalization

CAMOUFLAGING LIFELESS BLONDE HAIR

Rose's fine, limp hair looks broken, overcolored, underconditioned, and lifeless. If you have limp, dull hair, don't wear it combed straight down with a center part, a style that should be reserved for women with healthy, meticulously conditioned hair. And don't think you thin down your face by keeping your hair brushed down close to the sides of your head—it just drags you down, making you look washed out and older. The center part, especially, spells doom for thin, aging (remember, hair starts to age in your late 20s!) hair—this kind of part also exposes roots and regrowth too soon after your hair is colored.

In the afternoon, Terry Foster took Rose's damaged-looking hair in hand. The first problem: to keep as much *length* on very broken hair as possible. (Only one of the women pictured has short-short or pixie-cut hair. That's because when most women pass a certain age, they look better with some hair framing their faces. Besides, have you ever seen an over-30 pixie?) The solution: Blunt cut all the ends, which in turn thickens up thin hair. The shorter and longer strands were blended to give defined shape and style to the hair. The application of small rollers all over the head, each holding very fine sections of hair, produces the most possible wave and fullness, giving necessary movement to otherwise limp hair. The proportions of Rose's now full hair work with her body shape. The upswept, side-parted style gives a glamorous Marilyn Monroe look and counters the downward pull of gravity, which tugs against all our faces.

Rose's hair color, slightly warmed to a sunny honey blonde, is achieved with a single- rather than double-process coloring. If you have less than strong hair, it is more prone to damage now than it was when you were a younger, double-processed platinum blonde. (See the Time Machine photos and copy, following p. 194, if you are or would like to become a blonde.)

Step #3: The 29-and-Holding (Holding, Holding) Corrective Make-up Guide

How to make up to slim down a full face

Yesterday's young, round face can turn soft-looking when you pass 30. But you can "trick-slim" your face as well as your body. Actresses do it by creating high cheekbones where none exist via silicone implants (inserted in the gum area and tunneled up into the cheek region or put in place via the face-lift incision).

You can create your own face-slimming bone structure using less radical procedures. Your secret: cosmetic legerdemain.

℞. *To thin the top half of the face with color,* use blusher on outer forehead and high on cheekbones. Powder blusher placed as illustrated creates cheekbones; any look of prominent bone structure under soft, padded flesh will heighten the illusion of slimness. This color-framing technique also draws attention to the top half of the face (where there is less sag) and slims a broad forehead. A wide forehead further tends to round out the face.

℞. *To thin the bottom half of the face with contouring,* you must first learn the general contouring rules. Use a contouring product specifically made for shading. Regular blushers, even if they're brown or tan, have pink or orange undertones that make them unsuitable for the task at hand. (There *are* reasons why the industry makes a variety of products!) There are two contouring formulas.

Cream works best if your skin is very dry or if you're not that adept with make-up. You can move it around more easily than you can a powder, and you can blend it in more easily if your efforts result in too defined a look. (If contouring is not subtle, it can look ridiculous. Remember, the photography contouring worn by models and the street contouring you will use are two different things.)

Powder stays better, but be careful you don't overdo it. Once powder is applied, you will look smeared if you try to correct its placement with your fingers. Use a large, long-handled brush (not the little brush that comes with your blush compact) for greater leverage and control; skip the little brushes, as they aren't full enough to hold the amount of powder the sweeping motions of contouring require. When you use powder, blow on the brush after you "fill" it so there's almost no powder left to apply—this will insure a light touch.

Now that you know the whats, here are the hows to thin the lower half of the face.

Draw in your cheeks and pucker your mouth (so your face resembles a fish). Now, contour in the hollow beneath your cheekbones. Next, wrap the contour color from the hollow out to the side of your face right over your jawbone. This wraparound contouring "wraps up" what you don't want to show.

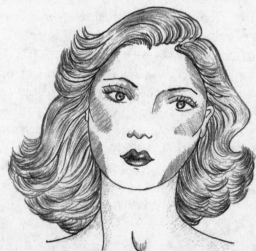

℞. *Use the eyebrows as frames.* If you have a round, full face, make sure your brows have a definite peak in them. The peak not only frames the eye attractively, it adds an angular line that your circular face needs.

℞. *Choose foundation with care if you have thin, fair skin.* If your skin is clear and fair, don't think you'll give yourself a porcelain look by choosing the lightest, whitest foundation you can find. Remember the shading rule: *Light emphasizes, darkness hides.* So if you're over 30, a very white foundation will only emphasize lines and wrinkles.

Instead, choose a make-up with a slight pink undertone. If you're very fair, a bit of rosy glow will help keep your face from disappearing into the woodwork.

Though you do want to add color, you don't want to add weight. If you have thin, dry skin like Rose's, a light soufflé make-up or cream make-up in a compact form will provide color, but not overpowering coverage, so your natural fairness will still shine through.

℞. *If you have good teeth, full lips,* and you are happy with the shape of your lips, outline with a lip brush, following your natural lipline, and fill in using a lipstick tube in the same color. If you're not as lucky as Rose, who has bright white teeth, you should avoid coral and brown lipsticks, which bring out the "yellow" in yellowing teeth (a common aging problem). Instead, use pinks or reds.

℞. *To bring out blue eyes, complement blonde hair,* don't use blatant, heavy colors. Rose's blonde hair and blue-red lips are giving a strong glamour message. When you were 21, you could pair these high-voltage effects with an equally powerful and sultry, devastating eye, but when you're 35-plus, a soft palette is more flattering, and it won't give you a "hard" appearance.

Light mauve tones and heathery lavenders work best. Because the colors are muted, you can completely surround your eye with color and you won't look as though you're overdoing it. Lavenders and mauves also serve as effective camouflage if you have thin, fair skin with little broken blood vessels showing through on your eyelids, because lavenders and mauves and broken blood vessels are in the same color family.

The color rule for every age, every eye color, is: If you wear shadow that matches the color of your eyes and is stronger in intensity, people will notice the shadow (which always looks deeper or brighter than natural color), and your own eyes will look insignificant by comparison.

℞. *To take away the "made-up" look,* consider a crushed pearl finisher, a highly pearlized cream formula you dot on forehead and high on cheekbones above blusher. The finisher gives skin a dry shine, a sheen like that of freshly scrubbed young skin. As you get older, it is important to wear make-up, but you want to maintain a *fresh*, polished look.

Step #4: Body Camouflage

BLACK MAGIC

The top Rose is wearing in the morning shot is too tight for her build. The close-fitting short sleeves emphasize a full upper arm (few of us who are less than young can get away with snug short sleeves). The necklace hits too low, exaggerating the chest; a loose, ill-fitting bra gives breasts a saggy look.

We purposely put Rose in clinging polyester pants (that show every bulge) to emphasize the saddlebag cellulite on the outside of her legs. Many women think pants hide everything, but unless they fit properly and are made of a firm material that will hang straight rather than hug every excess curve, the opposite is usually true. Poor posture is another youth-robbing negative.

The afternoon photo shows how Rose—and you, if you are her type—can look. I didn't perform black magic to create Option #2, but the wizardry does begin with a magical black dress. If your figure is such that you'll never be thin, use a black dress/suit to add glamour while slimming your silhouette. (Note: If you team black with no make-up and draggy hair, you'll only look glamorous to an undertaker. All the elements of your package must work together.)

The dress/jacket must fit loosely around the bustline. If a woman is both full-breasted and full-bodied she will give a more matronly appearance unless overly ample breasts are reduced by figure-skimming, loose-fitting clothes. A good bra is essential—an underwire or minimizer style will help firm and shape soft breast tissue. The breast area here is subtly defined by the high-cut square neckline, which shows pretty white skin and lengthens the neck (which is unlined and deserves exposing).

No pants for this figure. A straight sheath, fitting loosely around the derrière and thighs, creates a slender line. The slim, fitted jacket with long, narrow sleeves creates a long, slim-armed effect. The structured fabric caresses rather than clutches her curves; the jacket just skims the body, camouflaging a pot belly, spreading hips, and cellulite.

Need some holding in? Forget the girdle-girdle. If you don't want to look like your mother (you will in all-around paneling), try full-length support pantyhose. They firm up everyone's loose tummy, as well as tighten thighs. If you're not wearing a clingy knit, the support hose may be all the firming you'll need. A body stocking is a good alternative. Don't wear a long-line bra, especially under clingy clothes. The snaps and seams showing through will make you look as though your weight problem is out of control (and you'll also look old, old, old).

Color cue: If you're wearing black, use touches of color to add youth and spark to your outfit. Here, red does the trick in the dress; multicolored jewelry does the rest.

Step #5: A Little of the Young Razzle-Dazzle

COLORED STONES

You need not be a professional mathematician to learn an important 10-years-younger equation: *a touch of color = young*. Rose's necklace, set with red, green, and blue colored stones, reflects her "afternoon" fashion savvy. You *can* get a heady dose of color from rubies, emeralds, and sapphires. But if your gentlemen callers are more lavish with praise than trinkets, both color and quality can be had at a more moderate price with garnet (red), jade (green), or lapis lazuli (blue). All true gems are considered precious today, though their rarity places emeralds, rubies, and sapphires (diamonds, even colored ones, are not considered *colored* stones) in the ultra-precious category.

What should you consider when you're buying colored stones or *any* good jewelry? To help me give you the best technical information, I worked with the experts at Finlay Fine Jewelry—their jewelry is sold in major department stores all over the country.

The four main colored stone factors to consider are:

FACTOR #1: COLOR

Gemstones appear naturally in almost every color, and in a variety of shades, so you should be able to get a beautiful colored stone to fit your jewelry budget (but be realistic, we *are* talking about gems) as well as your taste. Color, and how it's distributed throughout the stone, is a prime factor in determining value. Stones with irregular coloring tend to be less expensive.

FACTOR #2: CLARITY

Light passes through a *transparent* stone as easily as it would through a glass of water. Through a *translucent* stone you see some light, but not clearly (the light appears to be filtered, as if you were looking at the stone through waxed paper); through an *opaque* stone there is no light pass-along.

FACTOR #3: CUT

Each of the three types of stones mentioned above is distinctive in its own way, and each must be cut to bring out its best features. A transparent stone is usually cut with *facets*, flat surfaces that allow light to enter the stone and be reflected back through the top. Translucent stones are usually cut *cabochon*—with a rounded, loaflike top surface (look at Rose's necklace). Opaque stones (moonstone, opal, jade, and turquoise are popular examples) are always cut cabochon. If you're looking at "cab" stones, remember that a highly rounded dome is considered more attractive than an almost flat profile. This is especially true if you're looking at "star" stones, cabochon-cut gems that appear to have six intersecting bands of light. The greater the depth, the more pronounced the star effect.

FACTOR #4: HARDNESS

Many women disregard this factor—to their ultimate disappointment. Some stones are more durable than others, and you don't want the jewelry you plan to wear every day to nick or scratch. When you choose your gem, ask your jeweler where it stands on the *Mohs scale*, an indicator of the relative hardness of the stone. A diamond, the hardest substance known to man, rates a 10; sapphires and rubies rate a 9; opals (more fragile stones) scale in at $5\frac{1}{2}$–$6\frac{1}{2}$.

Whatever kind of stone you buy, it's a good idea to ask if the stone or its setting needs any special care. Opals are a good example of a special requirement stone. They must be dipped in light mineral oil on a regular basis so they won't dry and crack.

You should also match your jewelry to your life style. If you love opals, but your job demands a lot of phone work, choose a pendant rather than earrings. And always keep harder stones separate from the more delicate softies in your jewelry box to prevent damage.

CHAPTER 15

🏵🏵🏵

The Over-30 Glamour Girl

Step #1: The Strategy

MAKE IT SEXY/KEEP IT CLASSY

In the morning picture Linda helped us to put together the "look style" of a woman who already envisions herself middle-aged, although she is only in her 30s. Her appearance is tidy, sensible—and drab. However she spends her time, she looks worn out from it. Her appearance does not give off young, happy vibes; it gives off stagnant, stuck-in-her-ways vibes.

If you see yourself the way we pictured Linda and you're trying to compete in the dating or working marketplace—you're not playing to win. You have to dress, look, and feel ready and able to beat the "kid" competition. That doesn't mean you put on the air of a young innocent. But you should heat up your image to give yourself a 10-years-younger, 10-years-sexier look and outlook—which doesn't depend on daytime cleavage and an 18-year-old body. It's far sexier to look worldly and sophisticated and very together, and that you can do for yourself.

My same-day strategy: Make every woman's fantasy become a reality. If you've ever been in the doldrums, what better way to lift yourself to a new high than to transform yourself into a glamour girl. As our afternoon picture shows, you needn't be (in fact you can't be) 18 to repackage yourself with sophisticated glamour.

Step #2: Hair Revitalization

SEXY HAIR

One thing is certain: You can't be glamorous with hair that's tidy and controlled, lacking freedom and style. Hair that is wrongly pulled back throws every facial flaw into harsh focus. If you have long, thick hair like Linda's, don't hide an obvious asset. Long hair always needs good shaping; if improperly cut, it just hangs there when let loose. If your hair is naturally oily, it needs washing often—a factor to be considered if you want to wear long hair. You must be willing to invest extra time in washing, drying, and care. Linda is. (So am I—I'm convinced that *long hair* is another way to spell *y-o-u-n-g*.)

Terry Foster reminds all of us to wear our hair to complement our personality, not our age. As you can see when Linda exercises Option #2, she really is young and vivacious and never should wear a matronly hairstyle (neither should you). By simply blunting the hair at the shoulders and layering it around the face, you can have a look that both frames and softens your face. *Soften* is a key word as you get older. Strategic layering and waving not only camouflages the beginning of jowls, it also serves two other purposes you may find helpful. 1) It lifts hair off the scalp, where oil collects. 2) By lifting the hair you give a needed lift to the face. When you're not 18, you can't have long do-nothing hair. It must be cut so that shape and style are built in.

Understand, too, that dark hair tends to make those first little wrinkles look more obvious. If you have long dark hair and a few lines, you, more than anyone, must make sure your hair is cut and shaped to wave around the face. The touch of softness will draw eyes away from tiny lines.

Step #3: The 29-and-Holding (Holding, Holding) Corrective Make-up Guide

HOW TO HIDE PUFFINESS

I'm a morning person—I work best early in the day, so that's when I schedule all of my important appointments. But lately when I wake up, I look puffy all around my eyes. *I* know that swollen look will disappear later in the day, but I can't announce to the people I'm meeting that my "condition" is temporary, so I've learned how to camouflage it.

If your face looks puffy, the cause could be water retention or allergy (see page 35), your period, too many glasses of wine the night before, certain medications (systemic cortisone, for example, or an unexpected reaction to antibiotics), or just the beginning of a change in facial contours that many women first experience when they hit their early 30s.

Here, ways to hide common puffy problems that can make you look older.

℞. *Consider pre–make-up "cold therapy" to reduce puffiness.* Get up three minutes early and apply an ice pack or the Swedish Freeze (page 72) to skin, or spray face with refrigerated mineral water. Keep your freshener or astringent in the fridge, and try keeping your (liquid) make-up base in "cold storage" also. If it doesn't thicken, the cool base will also help bring down the puffies a bit.

℞. *Give definition to a puffy face.* Since darkness hides, use a foundation one or two shades darker than your natural skin color. Stay in the warm beige family; it will blend best with your natural skin tone and you won't have any pink or orange undertones. Apply with a damp cosmetic sponge. The water on the sponge will thin out the foundation slightly; the sponge-as-applicator will help you blend the foundation properly (especially important if you're not matching your skin color exactly).

Deep-toned blusher properly applied also diminishes cheek puffiness, adds drama and glamour.

℞. *De-emphasize vertical nose-to-mouth expression lines* heightened by puffiness. If your vertical lines look like deeper shadows than they really are because puffy cheeks next to them create a stark contrast, run light blue cover cream down the nose-to-mouth creases and blend well to cast shadows away from this area. (Make corrections before you apply foundation.)

℞. *Hide first signs of incipient jowls.* If you have long hair, it's easy. Draw hair forward on your face.

℞. *Use shadow to conceal puffy eyes.* Swing your eye color palette over to the deep tones—sultry plum, smoky green, dark pewter, strong bronze. If your lids are unlined as Linda's are, choose cream, powder, or pencil—whichever you find easiest to work with.

Before applying eye make-up, make sure you understand eyelid anatomy (from the make-up artist's rather than the ophthalmologist's point of view). Your upper lid has three parts: 1) the *lid proper*, extending from the base of your lashes up to 2) the *lid crease or contour line*, where the lid indents, and 3) the *browbone*, the ridge above the crease that extends up to the eyebrow.

Because Linda has a small lid proper we put a light mauve on that area and we extended this lighter tone into her crease to open the eye a bit. (On a puffy lid the eye itself may look swollen closed—so some light shadow is crucial.) Darker plum is applied just above the crease and blended up and outward into her browbone region to help this puffy area recede.

℞. *Create stand-out drama.* If you've got great eyes (and you will get them when you learn how to do corrective make-up), rivet attention to them by rimming both upper and lower lids with black kohl pencil for all-out glamour. *How to:* Line around the outer two-thirds of both lids and smudge with your finger for a soft look. Don't completely encircle your eye with kohl—a full circle will close up the eye, making it look smaller.

℞. *Counteract the overhanging outer lid that puffiness produces* by using a *few* strategically placed false lashes, for *correction only*. The full-strip-of-lash look is out as fashion, but when I do professional make-ups, I see the difference a few correctly positioned lashes can make. Tiny clusters placed flush with the outer-corner lashes on your upper lid can give you that wide-eyed (not wild-eyed) look. The additional upsweep they provide gives your eye an upturned corner, a much younger look than the downward tug of gravity and time. Here's how to lash it for camouflage.

Buy an individual lash kit in a department or drug store. They're grouped in clusters of long and short hairs; pick what you need, and snip cluster off. (Since you'll be using only a few at a time, one kit should last you practically forever!)

Apply before rest of eye make-up to clean, dry lashes, and use only a powder (not cream) eyeshadow when you're finished.

Dip the tiny cluster into the supplied adhesive so that half of the lash is covered with glue.

Place lashes right up against your own lash (not lid), so three-quarters of your lash is covered, and pinch fakes against your own lashes.

To remove, dampen cotton pad with lukewarm water and hold against eye for 3 minutes. Remove pad, dip Q-tip into remover, and stroke eyelash with your eyes closed. Fakes will slip right off. Don't tug. You don't want to remove any of your own.

℞. *If you see a slight droop or puffiness around your mouth*, don't outline lips all the way into the corners. Jowls actually begin by your mouth (not by your jaw and chin, as many women think), and you don't want to draw attention to them.

Bonus: By ending the line just before the corners, your lips will appear to turn upward for a youthful, happy look. An upward tilt can change an unhappy, pouty mouth into a full, sensuous mouth.

℞. *To create a sensuous mouth, create a "spotlight" on your lips.* When you're filling in with color, a spotlight in the center of your mouth will draw attention to full, lush lips. Outline in a darker color and use that same deep tone to color in the entire upper lip, plus the outer two-thirds of the lower lip. Fill in the center of the lower lip with a lighter tone in the same family,

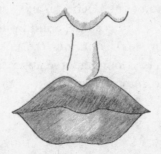

as illustrated. For example, you might outline in a mulberry and "spotlight" with a pinky mauve. Blend the two colors well. If the skin around your lips is unlined, like Linda's, gloss your entire lips for a moist, sexy look. But whenever you gloss, you definitely must outline your lips in pencil to keep the runny gloss from overrunning your mouth area.

Step #4: Body Camouflage

Getting that firm look

The body strategy: Give womanly, soft contours a young, *firm* look. To do it in a day with camouflage (while a diet and Body-Lifting produce long-term results), let's start by undoing some common errors Linda shows us. The shirt and skirt she's wearing in the morning are practical and conservative, but unexciting. The loosely fitting shirt covers Linda's thin waist, "wasting" a good feature; the short-cropped sleeve is a no-no for anyone over 30 who has more than a pound or two to spare—besides, the upper arm is an age giveaway on any woman. A washed-out, worn-out bra can make you look like a washout if you need some firming and uplifting (who doesn't?).

Linda's narrow waistline is further hidden by the skirt's matching tie belt, which does not cinch her waist. The loose extra fabric around the top part of the skirt adds pounds to already rounded hips. The entire outfit, besides providing no artful camouflage, is entirely too matronly.

The same afternoon Linda stepped before the camera giving off new vibrations—good-looking, sexy, youthful, with-it. With a change of clothes, she finally shed the age stereotype her hair revitalization and make-up corrections had begun to attack.

Her look is pulled together with a snug-fitting sweater that defines her slender ribcage and creates a slinky, long, and lean look. (A sweater always gives a young look.) A narrow, strippy belt pulled tight further emphasizes a small waist. The sweater is purposely long enough to cover ample hips; the slits at the bottom assure that there is no pulling around the hipline. The seven-eighth sleeve length cut wide at the bottom covers the top part of the arm, shows a slim lower arm and wrist. The open throat is sexy, but not blatant as long as cleavage is not too deep. An unpadded seamless underwire bra might be the best choice for Linda's figure and fashion.

A straight, narrowly cut skirt continues the firm and slim look downward, creating the impression of a long, tapered appearance.

Color cue: Muted classic colors in soft fabrics make Linda's message one of ageless glamour.

Step #5: A Little of the Young Razzle-Dazzle

ADORN YOURSELF WITH A GOOD WATCH

If you're a busy woman like Linda, who has a young neck that doesn't need much adornment, a good watch can be a better investment than lots of sparkle at the throat. When you buy a watch, you should consider it a fashion item that can enhance or detract from your overall "packaging." There are two status watches that are really timeless timepieces. The first is the black leather- or skin-banded Cartier tank watch, which can go from office to evening without interfering with any other jewelry you may be wearing. (It looks especially nice paired with a delicate gold bracelet, the way Linda is wearing hers.) The second is the gold or gold and silver flex-banded Rolex.

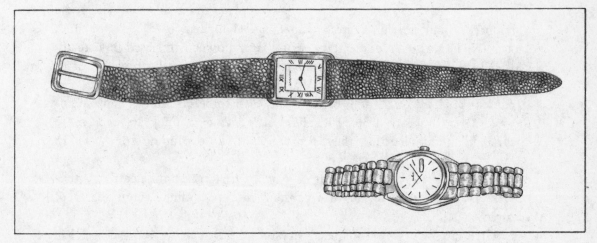

Both of these watches have at least one thing in common: They're very expensive. Luckily, there are less costly copies on the market that give off a similar well-dressed-watch look. The Cartier tank and Rolex gold *are* the top of the line. But there are other high-quality, elegant, and accurate tanks and real gold watches that are somewhat less expensive, and some copies are quite moderately priced. For example, you can get the Rolex "look" in gold or gold- or silver-toned metals. But if you're not comfortable wearing "fake gold," get a black leather–banded Cartier-style watch. Real leather isn't fake anything.

The two styles I'm suggesting both have traditional "hands" rather than a computer-type printout. When it comes to a classic watch, the less gimmickry the better. A day/date feature won't detract from the clean look of a timepiece, but if you also need to know what time it is in Japan, the depth of the ocean, or how fast you're running the mile, you need more than one watch.

Of course, you must consider more than style when you watch-shop. You also want accuracy. Buying a watch isn't as easy as it used to be. The following semi-tech language will help you understand what the salesperson is talking about.

Traditional jeweled watches. Small bearings of synthetic rubies are put into a watch to lessen friction (and the resulting damage) where one part of the movement rubs against another. A 17-jewel watch, therefore, has a jewel at each of the 17 points of greatest friction. Fewer than 17 jewels and you're not buying as durable a watch. More than 17 jewels isn't really necessary.

Pin-lever watches. Metal pivots replace the jewels. The pivots work well, but they don't last as long as jewels. These watches are lower in cost and may appeal to the woman who wants to build a watch wardrobe.

Electric watches use a small battery to replace the mainspring and some other parts found in the traditional mechanical movement. They are more accurate than a mechanical watch because their power is released in a steady flow. Electrics require no winding, but the battery must be replaced after about 12 to 18 months. (Most watch batteries cost only a few dollars.)

Electronic watches use a battery plus electronic circuits to replace additional parts of the traditional mechanical movement. They are even more accurate than the electrics; they also run without rewinding for 12 to 18 months (until the battery wears out).

Quartz crystal watches feature a battery that transmits electricity to a quartz crystal, which vibrates at a constant rate, providing a high degree of accuracy.

There are two types of quartz crystal *digital* watches. With the LED (light emitting diode) you have to push a button on the side of the watch case in order to read the time display. Battery life can be short, because each time you push the button to "read" the watch, energy is used up. Though many people like this kind of watch, I would find it inconvenient not to be able to see the time without freeing one hand to push a button. Besides, I think digitals look more like science fiction technology than jewelry.

The LCD (liquid crystal display) allows you to read the digital time without having to push any buttons. The numbers may (or may not) be artificially illuminated for night reading. Battery life is longer than with LEDs, lasting from 12 to 18 months.

The quartz crystal *analog* watch combines quartz technology with a conventional watch face, minute hand, and hour hand. Battery life is extremely long, ranging from one to five years, depending on the make of the watch. Many experts believe this will be the watch of the future.

CHAPTER 16

❦❦❦

From Early- to Mid-40s Grandma to Great Looking

Step #1: The Strategy

Update it/flaunt it

Judy is proud to be a chronologically young grandma (four times) who knows how to "keep it together," so she worked with me to show you what a "grandma" who *doesn't* work at her appearance can look like. Option #1, her morning mistakes image, is symbolic of the lack of positive packaging typical of so many women who have grown children and are divorced or widowed. Suddenly they're on their own, the perfect candidates for a mid-life rebirth, a second chance, but they don't know how to begin again. How many women in this position say, "If only I could look like I looked 10 years ago and know all I know now." Well, you can, as I'll demonstrate! Understand that commonsense good looks will help you get ahead in your job and get on with your life, but first you have to cut yourself free from that generation of women whose image stopped dead somewhere in the 1950s.

Everyone has seen women in their forties who seem afraid to change anything about their total "package" that will cut them off from the look they wore successfully when they were very young, at their most attractive (and possibly, happiest). If you fall into this "frozen looks" trap, understand that time has changed you physically, and by not changing your image from yesterday's to today's, you are making yourself appear older, not younger.

I devised a two-part strategy for women who share the problems Judy's

Option #1 symbolizes. First, you must leave behind those halcyon Eisenhower years and give yourself a contemporary, vigorous style that works today. Second, you must remember: If you've got it, flaunt it. Why hide a terrific slim body under a pile of years? With the right style and the right body you can wear almost anything, and believe me, you'll look right—not ridiculous. It's a matter of making sure all the parts work together to form a unified package whose individual components all give off the same message. In the morning photo, the *tried-too-hard, looked-too-hard* 1950s hair is at odds with a little nondescript dress—and the whole look adds at least 10 unnecessary years to Judy's A.M. persona.

Step #2: Hair Revitalization

CORRECTING TRIED-TOO-HARD, LOOKED-TOO-HARD HAIR

Long hair is not an error. The problem is long, *dated* hair. Judy's morning hairstyle is too designed, too plastered in place and old-fashioned looking. An Italian-boy top combined with a teased Suzy Parker flip doesn't work. (You can't have it both ways: Two hairstyles on one head is too much.) Don't try to frame your face by cutting short pieces of hair. An attempt to do for yourself what your hairdresser did 10 years ago is never successful. Besides, teasing equals freezing yourself into an old (and old-looking) image. The idea that framing the face will take off years is a sound one; here, it is the execution that's faulty.

Judy's hair color? She looks right as a blonde, but the morning roots show neglect and forget—it's every three weeks for a retouch.

Look at her afternoon picture—I love what we did to Judy's hair! The sleek look began with a fresh application of color to tone down her tried-too-hard blonde and conditioner to bring back sheen and elasticity to overbleached hair. (The longer you've been a blonde, the weaker your hair will be, so you must condition it regularly.)

As far as style goes, when you eliminate all the little doodads, you eliminate years from your overall look—and hours from your weekly hair-care schedule. Today's active woman cannot afford the time for a highly designed style. If you wear your hair the way we pictured Judy in the morning, you're probably a slave to a takes-forever hairdo. And when you're finished with all your hard work, your antiquated look will still miss by a decade.

The key: An ungimmicky, svelte hairdo to complement Judy's svelte body. Clean lines and graduated layering still frame the face softly, but now she has a totally contemporary look. Hair is artfully cut to expose beautiful youthful neckline and shoulders.

Step #3: The 29-and-Holding (Holding, Holding) Corrective Make-up Guide

How to cover flaws and erase years

Little problems become magnified without the proper use of make-up. Judy shows how you can hide these little flaws—and hide the years as well.

℞. *To camouflage broken blood vessels and adult messy skin,* apply tinted lavender underbase to block out ruddy skin tones produced by the appearance of broken blood vessels close to the surface as well as red "messy skin" bumps. Why *lavender?* Quite simply, it has the ability to neutralize other colors.

℞. *To further mask messy skin,* apply the foundation that will give you the necessary coverage. Teen-agers with skin problems use water-based make-ups. They can't use the heavier oil-based foundations because young people don't always clean their skin properly, and the oil in the make-up combines with the overabundant *natural* oils poor cleansing leaves behind to create further breakouts.

If you have *messy skin* and your skin is *normal to oily,* you clean it properly but you still don't want to compound the problem with an oil-based foundation, yet the water-based alternatives popular with teens won't give adequate coverage. The solution: a glycerine liquid powder foundation. This category contains no oil *or* water, yet it goes on wet and dries to a mat finish.

If your *slightly* troubled skin is *normal to dry,* you can use a cream make-up that comes in a compact to provide good coverage while adding a moist look to your face.

To be avoided: face powder. If you cover the more substantial foundation you need with powder, your make-up will look too thick and layered. (Besides, the glycerine liquid contains talc.)

℞. *To cover deep nose-to-mouth lines,* use a camouflage stick a few shades lighter than your foundation. These sticks usually come in convenient lipstick tubes, which you can stroke on over your lines and creases. But make sure your chosen stick is soft and moist enough to slide, not drag, across your delicate skin. If the formula is too dry, it may collect in lines, accentuating instead of hiding them. After applying, pat it into surrounding skin so it will blend well. (Look at Judy's afternoon pictures and you'll see how well this works.)

Alternate technique: If your dark shadows really bother you, go one correcting step further and buy an extra foundation a few shades lighter than your own. Pat lighter foundation over nose-to-mouth lines (as well as other obvious problem areas—vertical lines between brows, dark shadows under eyes). Always blend well.

When to do it: Whichever method you prefer, always cover specific flaws after you apply underbase, before you apply your allover foundation.

℞. *To camouflage a thin but loosening neck.* To mask the shadows that fall over your neck if it is thin and "cords" are beginning to stand out, blend a foundation one shade lighter than your own over the problem areas to cast shadows away from them. Bring face foundation over jawline and blend it with lighter-hued cord-camouflaging foundation color.

℞. *To perform brow-lift "face-lift."* You can take 10 years from your looks by giving the proper lift to your brows. Judy was wearing a thin, dark moon-shaped brow for our morning picture. Both the color and the shape are aging.

FOR PERFECT BROW COLOR

To add a lift to your face, you'll need two different brow pencil colors, one your true color and one lighter to create natural-looking brows. (Many companies make double-edged pencils in popular color combinations.) Just as the hair on your head is really different shades, so are your brow hairs.

If you're a blonde like Judy, you'll use a light blonde-colored pencil and scatter highlights in light brown.

If you have true red hair, you don't want red eyebrows. Your base color should be light brown; highlight with auburn, light or medium brown.

If you have soft red or light brown hair, choose a light brown brow color; highlight with medium brown.

If you have dark brown hair, use medium brown pencil and add dark brown highlights. (Dark brown alone looks too black, and black brows are a no-no for everyone.)

If you have gray hair, your base color will be light gray; highlight in medium gray.

FOR PERFECT BROW SHAPE

Don't draw your brow on in one stroke. You will do your brow one hair at a time (the way it really grows) using short, feathery strokes. Most of the "hairs" will be feathered on in your base color, with scattered strokes in your highlight color. The result will be a defined shape, but natural. I find it necessary to fill in my own brow shape with pencil. When thin brows were in style I tweezed mine into that barely-there look, but noticed (unfortunately) that brow hairs don't grow back quite as easily when you get older.

FOR THE PERFECT BROW-LIFT FACE-LIFT

Look at your own brows and consider the following.

Brows must arch up and out at outer corner. Brows that turn down at the ends make you look tired and unhappy, which in turn makes you look older.

If your brows are straight across, without any shape, they are not effectively framing your eyes. You need some arch.

Too-thin brows look sparse and old and must be thickened via feather-stroking with pencils (or brush—brow color also comes in brush-on kits).

Brows that are half-moon round will make you look as dated as Betty Boop.

Brows that grow thick, bushy, and untouched by tweezers need cleaning out. Scraggly-looking excessively haired eyebrows are not a sign of youth, just of laziness.

To recap: Until you see the difference the proper brow shape and color make, you have no idea how young a brow-lift can make you look. The guidelines are so simple: Your brows must turn up at the end, they must be drawn on in natural-looking feathery strokes, they must be lighter in shade than your own hair (unless you're a pale blonde) and they must be of more than one color.

Final Ŗ. *for brows:* No matter what shape you find most flattering, brush your brows up and out with a brow brush or old toothbrush for a younger, bright-eyed look.

Ŗ. *To create a more important frame for good teeth.* Judy has beautiful teeth, a young advantage, but her thin lips aren't a proper setting for these assets. Young equals full, especially in the mouth department. The technique for building full lips is described on pages 246–47, but if your thin lips (and your overall look) more closely resemble Judy's than Jan's, consider these two additional prescriptions.

Ŗ. *Color guide.* For Judy we used a plum-colored lip pencil and filled in with a plummy pink. If you find you look best in pink—and many blondes do—don't date yourself by wearing too pastel a shade. Instead, choose a pink muted with brown or plum for a soft but contemporary mouth.

Ŗ. *Don't cover your lips with gloss* if you have vertical lines around your mouth—gloss, which is very slippery, may actually leak into these lines. To get a shiny, glossy mouth (which is young-looking), I dot on gloss in the center of my bottom lip and blend it out just slightly so I have some *controlled* shine.

Step #4: Body Camouflage

SHOW IT OFF

Many women in their forties are concerned that they will look wrong in a slinky dress. Wrong! Not that you should go around in a micro-mini skirt just because you have good legs, but why hide a good thing? Rather, let Judy's afternoon picture be your guide to simple good-looks glamour.

Judy's covered-up morning dress did nothing for her: A nondescript dress creates a nondescript body, and the zipped-up, closed-off neckline hides some of Judy's best assets. Just because you're a grandma, you don't have to dress like yesterday's idea of the little old lady from Pasadena!

If you're over 40 and have a small bust, you're better off than large-breasted women. Your breasts won't hang so much, but they will lose their perky shape. In the morning pictures, Judy's bra does nothing for her. To create a firm-looking breast you might want to try a lightly lined fiberfill bra, or a plain knit with an underwire. For a hint of cleavage under low-cut dresses, a demi push-up bra or cups you insert yourself may be helpful. (You can also get a breast boost from your dress. Here the crisscross line across the breast gives a youthful lift.) An unstructured strapless bra allows movement while holding breasts *firmly* in place. (Bouncing breasts, small or large, are appropriate only for 18-year-olds or TV "sitcom" stars.) Of course, good posture picks up the breast while making everything else look younger and firmer. Slightly rounded shoulders will make even full, firm breasts appear to be concave.

Sophisticated T-shirt dressing is perfect for a slim figure of any age. Who says this inexpensive look must be reserved for the very young? Judy's "I've got it, I'll flaunt it" attitude shines through in this simple body-hugging style that emphasizes a slim frame, flat tummy, good unlined chest, and tight neck. She also shows off pretty shoulders and a slim, firm upper arm with her sleeveless look while her shiny patent belt draws attention to a slim waist.

Step #5: A Little of the Young Razzle-Dazzle

THE FOUR MUSTS . . .

With informal T-shirt dressing like this, you really don't need much in the way of jewelry. Judy is in such great shape that she is her own best adornment.

But if she (or you) were wearing more formal clothing and decided she really didn't have a thing (jewelry-wise) to wear, what would I suggest? If you're starting your good jewelry investments from scratch, I would recommend you buy the following, in the following order:

Must #1. A pair of small gold hoop, stud, or button earrings. The styles illustrated can be worn with almost anything.

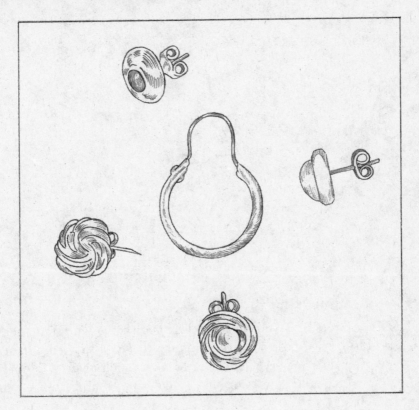

Must #2. One gold chain that can be worn with both high and low necklines. In time you can purchase one more, either longer or shorter, with a link style different from that on your first chain. (See the gold jewelry guide, pages 234–37, for a discussion of lengths, styles, karats.)

Must #3. A good watch. The two styles I recommend are discussed fully on pages 213–14.

Must #4. A small, interesting gold ring in either a simple geometric shape or a readily identifiable style such as Cartier's marriage band (a jewelry classic for many years), which is actually three interlocking bands. You can have it fashioned of pink, yellow, and white 18k gold, or all yellow gold. If you're not married, have it cut small enough to wear on your pinky.

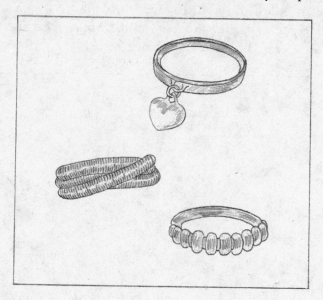

. . . AND FIVE WAYS TO GET THEM . . .

These four pieces of jewelry are simple enough to be worn together. But whether worn singly or ensemble, they signify that you're young, that you have a sense of quality and style, and more than a touch of class. Hopefully, you'll be able to keep adding to your jewelry collection. But before you make your first purchase:

Way #1. Study the editorial layouts in fashion magazines for an indication of jewelry as well as wardrobe trends. Look at the jewelry worn by the models in the magazine ads. Top clothing designers make certain their featured garments are paired with the right jewelry, and they hire expensive photo stylists to make sure everything works well together. Seeing how the pros put it together will give you an unerring feel for what goes with what.

Way #2. Deal only with reputable jewelers. If you haven't had much experience in this area, the jewelry sold in a good department store may be your best bet, because what is sold there is backed by the store's reputation.

Way #3. Ask a friend whose jewelry you admire where she shops, especially if you're interested in redesigning an old piece you already have.

Way #4. Don't just look at the piece you like in the case and say, "I'll take it." Ask to try it on to see how it fits with your face and body; study the jewelry in a mirror as you're wearing it. (Of course you won't be allowed to stroll away from the jewelry counter! The better the merchandise, the tighter the security.)

Way #5. Develop a relationship with one good jeweler. If you buy a few pieces from the same jeweler, he *may* loan you the jewelry you *think* you love to live with before you buy it. In this way, you won't make an expensive mistake, and wind up with a ring, necklace, or whatever that never sees the light of day (or night).

. . . AND THIRTEEN WAYS TO COMMUNICATE WITH YOUR JEWELER . . .

If you're ready to shop for your "Musts"—or any good jewelry—you'll find it helpful to understand the terms that indicate how jewelry is crafted and finished. I do think that when you're planning to buy anything, you get better service—and a better understanding of what you're paying for—if you can speak the vocabulary of the people you're dealing with.

Here, a baker's dozen of terms that *won't* turn you into a lapidary (person who fashions stones), but will give you a little more knowledge than the average lay shopper.

- Satin—a finish with a soft, pearllike luster instead of a bright polish. The polish is dulled by scratch-brushing, sandblasting, or chemical treatment.
- Highly polished—the metal has been buffed to a bright, shiny finish.
- Florentine—meshlike finish with crisscross texture; the metal is actually cut into to achieve this finish.
- Hammered—finish produced by banging a number of tiny dents into the metal's surface.
- Engraving—sharp tool used to cut out a design. Metal is actually cut away. It can be used to outline a design, cut out figures, or produce letters.
- Chasing—an ancient art of decorating metal by hand with figures or ornamental patterns. It differs from engraving in that chasing "flows" the metal into raised or indented decorations, using hand hammers and punches of various sizes and types.
- Antiqued—finished to have an appearance of old age.
- Cloisonné—thin strips of metal are attached in the form of a design to the surface of a piece of metal. The spaces enclosed by these wire strips are filled with different colors of enamel.

□ Enameling—pulverized glass that produces a wide variety of colors is applied to the surface of metal or glass; the piece is then baked in an oven (in less expensive enameled jewelry, the enameling is simply painted on, not baked). Note: Enameling chips easily; be careful with enameled jewelry.

□ Cameo—figure carved from shell or colored stone; the carved figure is above the surface.

□ Intaglio—part of the stone is carved out; the design lies below the surface.

□ Inlay—small, flat pieces of metal, such as gold, or pieces of stones are set into a piece of metal or wood in a decorative design.

□ Findings—premanufactured small parts (catches, links, settings), used in jewelry production.

CHAPTER 17

❦❦❦

Career Dressing:
Mock Man . . . or Dynamic Woman?

Step #1: The Strategy

INDIVIDUALIZE IT

Margarita is a young career woman. In her morning photos she and I give
you our interpretation of the "mock man" dress code. Many women feel
that a uniform based on a severely tailored suit (and hair either severely short
or unfemininely pulled back) will help them climb the ladder of success.

Ridiculous! This "uniform" look ages the young woman pictured. She
is only 25, yet her morning image reverses everything youth has going for
it. In the A.M. her presentation is so stiff, formal, and serious that she adds a
decade to her looks.

There is nothing "wrong" with a tailored black suit, but it's certainly
not the necessary uniform for everyone who works. What is wrong (and a
shame) is that so many young Margaritas let stereotyped, misguided rules of
business decorum cow them into unconsciously substituting average dull-
looking replacements for girls who have the potential to be great-looking.

Our strategy: Take Ms. Young Businesswoman out of an unbecoming
masculine-oriented uniform and show her how to look and dress like the
beautiful individual she is. We wanted to prove that a woman can dress
dynamically and in good taste—and still look like a woman.

Step #2: Hair Revitalization

Businesslike needn't be boring

Margarita's morning hair is the extreme of no-style conservatism. The pulled-back look does nothing for her even though she has a young face. (Whether you're 15 or 50, don't wear your hair off the face if the style shows your ears to a disadvantage.)

Many women make the mistake of assuming pulled-back hair is a time saver, but a good haircut and the basic hair-setting procedure you learned in Part Five will not only help you look successful without too much fuss, it will also save your hair (even if you wear coated elastic bands, all that pulling on the hair day after day is sure to cause breakage, which in later years will contribute to a look of allover thinning hair).

Terry's suggested cut for Margarita's hair: a style suitable for a young woman who wants to look both daytime glamorous and career serious. By keeping as much width as possible at the outer edges of the hair (to frame the face) and removing some weight throughout the crown to produce a look of varied lengths, your hair will move when you do. The afternoon picture shows hair that is softly long and feminine, but appropriately styled for every business environment.

Margarita's hair color is perfect for her complexion. But what changes should you consider if you're a 35-year-old (or 45+) brunette? Turn to the Time Machine, page 259, and see what a difference the years may make.

Step #3: The 29-and-Holding (Holding, Holding) Corrective Make-up Guide

How to make up for success

If you're a success-oriented young working woman, your total package must include more than cursory attention to make-up. Here are skin and make-up corrections for the woman on her way up.

R. *To compensate for an oily adult complexion.* If you're a busy woman whose oily skin "breaks through" your make-up, you'll get a tired, messy look that says the day is over—even though it may only be 11 A.M. To compensate, wear a long-lasting glycerine liquid powder foundation. Because it provides coverage without oil, your make-up won't turn orange (or invisible) as the day wears on. I wear this type of make-up because it eliminates the need for frequent touchups, a time luxury I can't afford.

If your oily skin is accompanied by now-and-then breakouts, or if you have one annoying blemish you want to get rid of fast and sensibly, carry a blemish stick with you (many companies make them) so you can (and should) dab it on the affected area several times a day over your make-up.

℞. *Consider face powder*, a great help in controlling excess oil. Many sold today are called "wet" powders (look for one that says it contains a moisturizing agent); they don't give you an old-fashioned cakey-powdery look . . . they just set your make-up. Powder is essential if you live in a hot, humid climate that seems to peel the make-up from your face as soon as you step out the door. (Hot weather causes your foundation to sweat right off.)

To apply powder, use a brush for even, controlled distribution. Fill the brush, then blow or shake the excess off before dusting lightly across your face. (As much should wind up in the air as on your face. You don't want a *heavily* powdered look.)

Exception: Glycerine liquid powder foundation contains talc, so you wouldn't powder over it.

℞. *For hyperpigmentation* (*brown patches*). While speaking with Margarita, a Miami resident, about some complaints that face women in hot climates (heat causing make-up to "sweat off" and disappear, for example), I thought of another problem that sometimes bothers sun-country residents: light and dark pigmentation patches on the skin (which can also be caused by pregnancy or the Pill). I see many young women (usually the olive-skinned) with this problem. If you can't avoid the sun completely or you have hyperpigmentation problems from another cause, consider the following cosmetic camouflage suggestions:

If you have oily skin and quite noticeable pigmentation, try a glycerine liquid powder foundation over a tinted underbase. Together they will help mask out unwanted color, thus evening out skin tone.

If you have dry skin with noticeable pigmentation, pair your underbase with a cream foundation.

If you have minor pigmentation problems and not much else in the way of blemishes, you can wear a thin, whipped soufflé make-up over your tinted underbase. When you add an underbase to your make-up ritual, you don't need a heavier foundation. Sometimes using more than one product can give you a *less* made-up look. Choose your soufflé in a shade one tone darker than your natural skin color to blend in with hyperpigmented areas.

℞. *Make-up for success*. Margarita's afternoon make-up is perfect for a dynamic career woman. If she stands up to make a presentation, you can be sure she will receive complete attention. Remember, it's not only what you say or how you say it, it's how you *look* when you say it.

Wear powerful colors that complement your natural coloring; apply them with strong, deft strokes. Your make-up should be as carefully planned as your clothing.

Understand that powerful make-up doesn't mean thick, heavy make-up. It means creating a confident image by wearing the right amount of make-up applied in just the right way.

Margarita wears clear, definite red lipstick to call attention to a strong mouth, and rust-red blusher to counteract her olive-tending-to-sallow skin.

"Success" eyes are lined with a brown-black pencil both top and bottom, starting from the center and working to the outer edge, and the top lashes are mascaraed. Direct and on-target eyes will mesmerize a business meeting —but this is the *only* intense eye make-up you will wear. Leave your "the eyes that launched a thousand ships" palette for other occasions. Ms. Career Woman's eyes are shadowed here in soft beige and brown tones. Yes, Margarita would also look terrific in a wide range of colored shadows, but these more flamboyant shades would detract from the businesslike image she is trying to project.

℞. *If you're planning to go out straight from the office* and you don't have time to stop home first, it would probably be inconvenient to scrub your face and start making up from scratch. (There's no place more crowded than the office ladies' room at 5:01 P.M.) Instead, go day-for-night at your desk (you do keep a magnifying stand-up mirror in your drawer, right?) by applying your evening look *right over* your daytime cosmetics. Here are four make-up—intensifying steps that will take just 5 minutes!

Step #1: Reapply your lipstick and add a shimmery pearl gloss in the center of your lower lip for a bit of night shine.

Step #2: Brush on a pearlized blusher one shade deeper than your no-pearl daytime color.

Step #3: If you're wearing muted eyeshadows, sweep across lid with a metallic glitter shadow in the same family—metallic copper would work over a daytime beige.

Step # 4: Add more mascara—three coats. For evening, don't forget your bottom lashes.

Step #4: Body Camouflage

DRESS YOUR BODY LIKE A WOMAN'S

The non–figure-forming unrelievedly black suit Margarita wears in the morning makes her look as though she's in mourning! The loose-fitting jacket and prim and proper blouse give no indication of the terrific young body to be found underneath all that drab.

The afternoon picture shows a dynamic, well-dressed young woman. I have showed the extreme—a fire-engine-red silk dress—to prove that there is nothing wrong (and everything right) with looking like a glamorous working *woman*, if you do it in good taste. The dress has a daytime neckline and A-line skirt that moves with the body without overpowering it. If you are going to wear feminine, soft dresses by day, be careful that the skirt isn't billowingly full (you don't want to look as though you're ready for the cocktail hour at 10 A.M.).

Of course, even an attractive woman like Margarita wouldn't make a red silk dress the staple of her business wardrobe, but by showing you that even properly cut red silk can be right, I wanted to prove that a woman needn't appear day-in, day-out in a grim, mannish suit to be taken seriously.

This is not to say that I'm not a fan of the well-suited look. A terrific-looking suit (or suits) should be an important part of your business wear, but you don't want to look nose-to-the-grindstone just because you're in an office. Here's what you need to know to invest in a suit that will make you look like a million while you're out there *earning* that first million.

SUIT UP WITH STYLE

℞ #1. *Don't be afraid of color.* A well-cut, very tailored suit needn't be black or navy. Mulberry, deep green or (yes!) red will keep you looking feminine, and soften the harsh edges.

℞ #2. *The cut of the jacket* is the most important feature. If you can afford just one good suit, make sure it features a single-breasted blazer—the most classic cut of all. If it's a tweedy or solid blazer, you can pair it with other skirts as well. A blazer worn over any well-cut skirt gives a "suited" feeling, and an unmatched suit is stylish.

A single-breasted blazer has another point in its favor besides classic good looks: You can wear it open or closed. A double-breasted jacket looks sloppy worn open; a belted jacket looks odd worn open for daywear—it must be properly cinched to give a businesslike look.

Be careful when you buy a short-jacketed suit. A short jacket, especially double-breasted, can be stylish but it's not as versatile. You can't always wear it over other skirts—it may not work with fly fronts, dirndls, pleats. The cropped jacket is usually cut to fit the specific skirt it is paired with. I learned this lesson when I bought an expensive short-jacketed suit with the idea I could wear the jacket with just about anything. Well, it didn't work out that way!

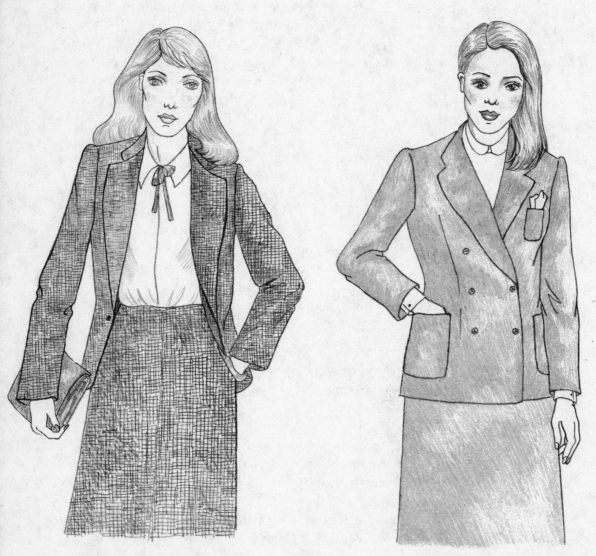

SINGLE-BREASTED BLAZER   DOUBLE-BREASTED BLAZER

But if you already have your basic blazer look, you should add another suit with a slightly less traditional cut that could only be worn by a woman. The four suit looks pictured won't make you look as though you're wearing a uniform—you'll just look right, and ready for promotion. You'll notice we don't illustrate the hemlines, which go up and down as fashion changes, because the jacket is the focal point of a good suit.

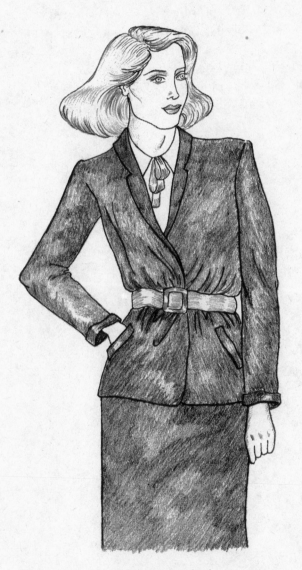

BELTED WRAP JACKET

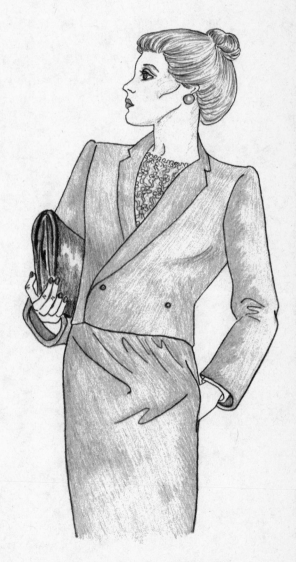

CROPPED DOUBLE-BREASTED JACKET

℞ #3. *Invest in good fabrics.* Good wools, tweeds, and gabardines are not inexpensive, but they pay for themselves by helping to give you a successful, polished image. Try to invest in seasonless fabrics. A lightweight wool, for example, can be worn in spring or fall, as well as winter.

℞ #4. *Flash colorful accessories.* A toned-down, no-nonsense suit should be livened up with touches of color—either in your shirt or sweater, neck scarf or jewelry.

℞ #5. *Think evening before you buy.* It is possible for a very tailored suit to make the transition to "after 5" successfully. Shown are two ways to dress up the tailored wrap jacket.

Evening option #1: A wider, fancy belt in either suede or a fabric other than sporty leather gives a night look. So does trading your daytime blouse for a simple camisole, a garment so easy to make, you might try sewing one

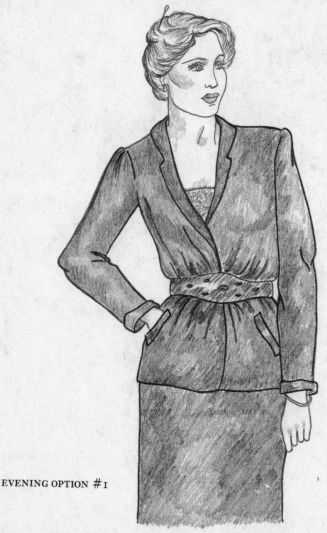

EVENING OPTION #1

up yourself in a dressy fabric (lace adds a feminine touch) or asking a dress-maker to custom-make one for you if you can't find the color/style that would best transform your favorite suit from day to after dark. An upswept hairstyle, hair ornament, and simple jewelry complete an "after 5" look perfect for cocktails or dinner.

You're going to a really gala event straight from the office? Consider *evening option #2.* The important changes here: The wrap jacket is left open, revealing a fancy, beaded camisole with spaghetti straps. Consider bugle beads or sequins, silk or satin, for all-out glamour . . . and consider yourself well dressed for a night on the town (without the inconvenience of stopping home to change first). More prominent formal jewelry also adds to the "big night" look.

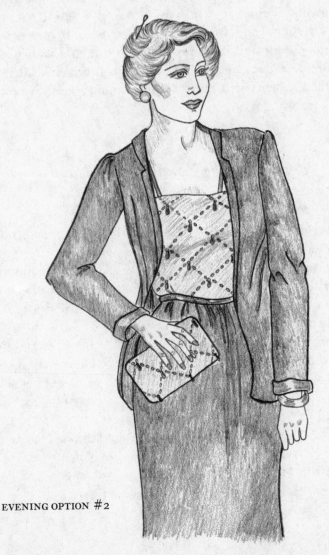

EVENING OPTION #2

Footnote: Naturally, you'll need a change of shoes and bag to complete an evening look.

℞ #6. *You'll never totter to the top!* You've paired a great suit with uncomfortably high heels? If the heel height of the moment is too high for you to walk comfortably and authoritatively, it's better to come down a notch in shoe height than detract from the self-confident, dynamic image only a steady gait will provide.

Postscript

I recently was asked by a group of businessmen if I would invest my money with a woman stockbroker who was wearing a sexy see-through blouse and no bra. Of course not! I would not invest with *anyone* who did not appear to have good sense and show proper judgment. If a woman could not make a more sensible decision concerning proper business attire, she would not use good judgment with my money. Common sense is common sense, no matter what the situation.

Step #5: A Little of the Young Razzle-Dazzle

A GUIDE TO BUYING GOLD JEWELRY

The simple pearl pin and earrings further add to the subdued, nondescript, and matronly mood befitting Margarita's morning option.

Margarita's afternoon jewelry is much more casual and contemporary. When you look terrific and you're wearing a vibrant color, you don't need expensive glitter. We put frankly costume jewelry on Margarita to show that you don't always need the real thing to look right.

But as any young career woman advances, she'll want to start buying better jewelry—and the best place to start is with gold. While it may be comforting to have some Krugerrands stockpiled in a Zurich bank, gold as adornment is more fun, and since the price often changes, you may convince yourself you're buying gold jewelry as a hedge against inflation! One of the best places to shop for exquisite gold jewelry is a reputable coin dealer. Many gold coins and pieces have exquisite designs. Whether you prefer the 20-dollar American eagle, a Mexican 50-peso coin, or a Swiss ingot, you'll have a piece of "jewelry" that is both valuable and timeless.

After your purchase, bring your gold piece to a jeweler to be framed, and pick out a gold chain that will best set it off. When times are good, you can border the coin with stones if you wish; if times are bad, you can always remove the coin from the frame and resell it—just make sure no holes are drilled into it when it is first set and/or adorned. "Coin of the realm" can also be used for earrings, bracelets, belt buckles.

With or without a gold piece pendant, gold chains look terrific on everyone. If you're wearing more than one, remember all chains should hit above or below your breast, never right at your bustline (especially if you're large-breasted). The classic styles are the S-chain, rolled snake chain, and link type. All come in a variety of lengths and weights. The 15-to-16-inch choker that fits loosely around the neck is the most popular because it's the least expensive. The other classic lengths are 18 inches (princess); 24 inches (matinee); 30 inches (opera or double choker). Which you buy depends on your budget and your body (you want the chain to hit or miss your bust at the most flattering angle).

If you're thinking of switching your jewelry to the gold standard, you must understand what *karat* means. Pure gold is 24 karat, and is easily scratched and dented, so it is rarely (if ever) used for jewelry; 14 karat gold jewelry means that 14 parts out of 24 are pure gold. The additional 10 parts are a metal added to strengthen the gold. Jewelry may be marked from 8, 9, 10 karat to 14, 18, 22 karat. The higher the karat, the more expensive the jewelry.

The different colors of gold depend on which strengthening metal is used. Copper imparts a reddish glow, silver a greenish cast. Together, the addition of copper and silver produces a white gold.

If you buy gold abroad, the karat will be noted in decimal form: 18k gold jewelry would be marked .750, because it is ¾ ($^{18}\!/_{24}$), or 75 percent, pure gold. The colors of gold differ according to the tastes in different countries. In the United States, 14k yellow gold (called Hamilton color by jewelers) has been the traditional favorite, but 18k is catching up. Recently, with gold prices flying about, 10k gold has been gaining more fans. (Often, economy influences fashion.) On the international scene, Italians like 18k green or yellow gold; 18k pink or white gold is favored by the French and Germans, while 18k yellow holds sway in South America.

Gold-filled jewelry is less expensive because only ½₀ of the item must be pure gold. The gold is fused to a base metal in the filling process. If a 12k piece of jewelry is involved, the marking might read ½₀ *12k G.F.* (gold-filled).

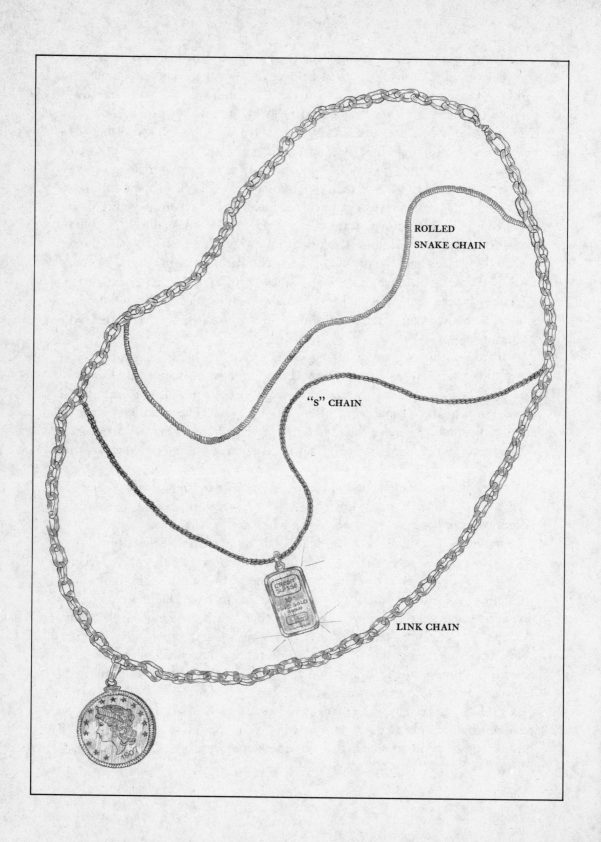

ROLLED
SNAKE CHAIN

"S" CHAIN

LINK CHAIN

Gold-plated is the least expensive piece of "gold" jewelry you can buy. Extremely thin layers of gold (measured in microns) are flashed on a base metal via electricity. The more layers of gold, the more expensive the piece of gold-plated jewelry. Plating is noted as *G.E.* (gold electroplate) or *H.G.E.* (heavy gold electroplate).

CHAPTER 18

❦❦❦

Life Begins at 40

Step #1: The Strategy

ENERGIZE IT

So many women in their 40s today are ready to start a new life. But whether they're divorced and want to wipe the slate clean, are looking for a career the second time around, have waved bye-bye to their children, or are just plain bored-bored, they won't be able to change anything if they don't change their appearance first. Patricia and I created two image options for you, but there's only one choice. No matter where you want your turning point to take you, if you look old, you'll feel old, and if you look young, you will feel young. If you see a little of yourself in the morning photo, follow our strategy: Give yourself a shot of youth by energizing your appearance.

Step #2: Hair Revitalization

GIVING SHORT HAIR YOUNG STYLE

In the morning photo, Patricia's hair, matronly and dreary in both color and style, is as tired looking as the rest of the look she represents. Keeping your hair short to maintain a youthful look is not enough when it's teased and styled carelessly. Adding a brown color rinse over graying hair produced a drab, mousy effect, giving hair a discolored instead of gray-covered cast—remember, temporary rinses don't do much.

In the afternoon we recut her already short hair into a definite style easily maintained. Since uplift is so important with the years, we brushed her hair up to pull up her features. Softness is left at the neck so the look isn't harsh. In Patricia's case, with her potential for long, lean good looks, short and sleek is actually more appropriate than face-framing fluffy. Just look at her afternoon hair—living proof that an energized blonde can have more fun than a mousy-looking, washed-out, no-color brown-haired woman.

Step #3: The 29-and-Holding (Holding, Holding) Corrective Make-up Guide

How to do away with sallowness and uneven skin color, undereye circles, dark-pigmented lips and eyelids

℞. *Neutralize sallowness.* Sallow skin tone is a big problem as we get older because our circulation is more sluggish, so it no longer brings the color to our cheeks as it did in the first bloom of youth (and we don't even embarrass easily anymore—so we can't rely on blushing to help!). Chapter 2 tells you how to improve circulation and natural color internally, but why not let make-up give Nature an honorable boost, in the form of a tinted underbase to strip out unattractive color and give your skin a "porcelain" canvas. A lightweight underbase (called a toner by some manufacturers because it evens out splotchy skin tones) also provides a thin cover over fine lines. An underbase solves many different skin problems. Besides blocking out muddiness, pigmentation problems, and blemishes, it masks the yellowish tinge so characteristic of sallow skin.

℞. *Camouflage dark circles under eyes.* For very dark circles (often caused by heredity, so even if you lead a monastic existence, they won't go away), a lighter color foundation applied under the eyes just isn't enough. When you first apply your make-up in the morning, use a light blue cover cream rich in oils. Light blue casts shadows away from the face (a trick first discovered by television studio make-up artists), turning dark areas into light. You will only have to put one layer of foundation over the blue to achieve a finished, shadow-free look, whereas if you relied on a lighter color and weight of foundation for coverage, you would need a few layers—which would look thick and unnatural under your eyes.

For during-the-day touchups (which may be necessary because the undereye often gets a tired, worn-out look), carry a camouflage stick for repair work. The stick must be a lighter shade than your foundation (but not so light you look owl-eyed), and it must be wet enough to glide across your skin easily.

℞. *Camouflage dark-pigmented eyelids.* Some women look like they're wearing dull, drab, unbecoming eyeshadow when they're not! I see this problem on many women when I do my promotional tours. Luckily, it is easy to correct.

Fight this darkness by using a cream specifically designed as an eyeshadow base. Because these lid foundations (almost every cosmetic company makes them) are creamy, they won't settle in tiny cross-hatched lines the way a powder would, and their "nude" color serves two purposes. 1) It lightens your natural lid color, keeping the lid from muddying up your chosen shadow shade, and 2) it allows you to apply eyeshadow more sparingly (there's no dark color to hide) so you won't need thick applications of color that will collect in creases.

℞. *Hide the beginnings of a double chin.* Yes, it happens to thin women in the form of empty-looking sag (on heavy women it looks like an extra fat pad). To counteract it, you must contour this area. Sweep your contour-

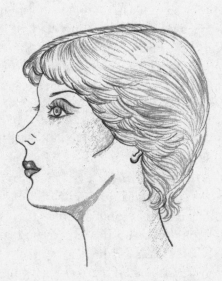

ing agent on a line just under your chin from one jawbone to the next and blend well. The slight darkness will make a tending-to-sag chin recede.

℞. *Camouflage naturally dark-pigmented lips.* When you were young, your lip color may have resembled lush ripe cherries; now, your lips look bluish (the way children's do when they've stayed in the pool too long)?

To lighten up your lips and your looks, use a lip stabilizer, a staple in most cosmetic lines. These gold-colored lipsticks hide the natural lip color, keeping that blue tinge from showing through. They're essential for anyone who has a problem with lipstick changing color, because they insure that your chosen lipstick shade won't be dulled or drably darkened by your own dark-pigmented lips. I use a gold stabilizing lipstick under my lipstick because it helps the color stay on longer, so it keeps my lipstick looking fresh longer. When your lipstick starts wearing off, you take on a worn, tired look (which translates into "older").

℞. *Give your face a youth transfusion via color.* If you don't have that healthy, outdoorsy pink-cheeked and clear-eyed look, don't go out of the house until you give your face a shot of badly needed cosmetic color. Without it, you'll be just another drab (rather than pretty) face.

Once you've masked out the shadows, you can subtract 10 years by adding life-giving color to your face. Look at Patricia in the morning and afternoon, then look at yourself with and without color. *Every woman over 30 needs blusher. Every woman over 30 needs lipstick. Every woman over 30 needs mascara.* (Soft-colored eyeshadows, though not essential, also make a tremendous difference.)

℞. *Give your cheeks a shot of color and re-create the visible cheekbones that will counteract a starting-to-slacken face.* Your cheekbones *are* still there, it's just that when you pass 30, they lack the definition very young, super-firm skin imparts.

To rediscover the bones, first you must find them. Break into a smile. The center fleshy "apple" part of your cheek is where you applied blusher when you were a young girl. Now, you have to place color a little differently to re-create that high-boned look. I showed you how to make cheekbones if you're a powder fan in "From Supermarket to Superwoman"—here I show you how to do it with liquid or cream. Apply 4 dots of color (page 242). Only the first dot is dead center on your "apple." Notice that the top dot is on a line just above the top of your brow; no dots are in the crow's-feet region because color gravitates toward lines. If you have crow's-feet or a real sunburst around your eyes, you certainly don't want these lines highlighted with moving cheek color. Instead, blend color out to hairline.

In Patricia's afternoon picture, she has the high-cheekboned look she

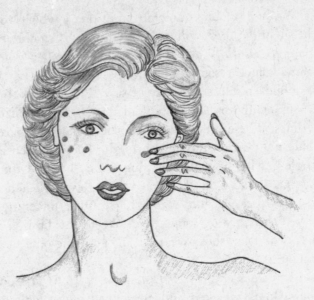

enjoyed 10 years ago. Who's to say if it's real . . . or make-up? (And, who cares!)

Step #4: Body Camouflage

How to emphasize a tall, lean figure

The boxed-jacket, ill-fitting navy blue suit lacks pep and gives a "matron in a women's prison" look. The entire outfit becomes a drab cover-all, and Patricia's figure does not need to be hidden. Even her circle pin is clasped in an out-of-date fashion.

In the afternoon, you can see how Patricia's tall, lean figure can be shown to advantage in well-cut, slim pants that fit snugly over her small rear; panty briefs rather than bikinis or hip-huggers will assure that there are no bumps and bulges to mar the sleek, long-legged effect. (If your derrière is flat, remember to round it a bit with briefs that have a seam running up the back—seaming adds definition.) Backless black patent leather shoes add just the right fashion touch to this pants look.

Up top, Patricia wears a snug-fitting black shirt and a turquoise polished cotton jacket cinched with a wide belt to show off her small waist.

Doesn't her afternoon fashion picture exude energy? It looks as though Patricia had a 10-years-off shock treatment! But the "shocking" difference comes in large part from bold use of color—from her hair and face to her turquoise top.

Step #5: A Little of the Young Razzle-Dazzle

THE FRANK FAKES

There is a definite place for costume jewelry in every woman's wardrobe. Frank fakes allow you to add a trendy note to your packaging that will update whatever you're wearing. Fakes also allow you to indulge your jewelry whims and fancies, without having any morning-after regrets that you spent your savings on something that will be as out next year as it is in this year.

There is just one rule that applies when buying costume jewelry: *Don't try to be the great imposter*. Make sure the piece that catches your eye looks costumey rather than imitative of precious jewelry. Frankly fake makes much more sense than almost real.

The yellow "artsy" bird pendant hung from a black cord in Patricia's afternoon picture adds fun and a bit of the unexpected to her outfit. It also conveys a subliminal message: This woman has a lively, young, unique personality.

Other good possibilities in the costume jewelry department include shells, art deco plastic, wood, crystal, beads, mock coral, Lucite, brightly colored plastic bangles, rhinestones that don't look as though they're trying to pass for diamonds, feathers, colored glass, leather, bone, heavy metal.

CHAPTER 19

☙☙☙

Mommy, Is That You?

Step #1: The Strategy

Unrealistic? then forget thinny-thin

In the A.M. photo, Jan helped me to symbolize for you the look of a woman who finally pulled through the child-rearing years. You can almost hear the woman with this look style say:

"I gained this weight finishing the kids' leftovers."

"I wore my hair exactly like this the very evening Daddy proposed to me."

"I've been so busy car-pooling and keeping the house that I had no time to myself."

Well, the kids do finally grow up, your husband does get promoted, your interests and values do change with time, and so must you. The empty nest syndrome happens to so many women. If your children have flown off, go back to work, back to school, back 10 years.

The strategy: to deal successfully with a body that will never be model-thin, except possibly through more effort than mere mortals are willing or able to make. If you have a never-skinny body, you're dieting and exercising to firm and lift what you can't lose. Now you'll learn the camouflage tricks that will help you forget thinny-thin and appreciate your own special look.

The sub-strategy: to show women how to soften that which has become dated and hard looking through abuse or neglect.

Step #2: Hair Revitalization

SOFTENING AN "ERECTOR SET" HAIRSTYLE

The main hair mistake Jan portrays for you: a belief that curls piled on top of the head add height and make the face look thinner. In reality, this style does nothing but accentuate the worst of everything. Wearing an "erector set" hairdo year in, year out means hair must be constantly teased and coated with hair spray to maintain its shape. This overkill contributes to faded, abused hair that must be cut off.

To turn around hair like Jan's, Terry suggested a layered, permed look. No light body wave, but a real perm that gives definite curl and shape to the hair. With this style, you can just towel-dry your hair and use an Afro-pick to lift it away from the scalp, fluffing your hair into the soft face-framing style in which it is cut. Her hair looks clean and healthy, and no hair spray is required. To give a further hair- (and therefore face-) lift, a nonperoxide soft brown hair color will bring back the warmth, lights, and life lost through years of hair abuse.

Step #3: The 29-and-Holding (Holding, Holding) Corrective Make-up Guide

HOW TO DO A THIN, SHEER, ALMOST INVISIBLE MAKE-UP ON THIN, BEGINNING-TO-LINE SKIN

Some women look best when they look as though they're wearing no make-up at all, either because they present a healthy, outdoorsy "package," they're older, or they have that thin English-Irish-Scottish skin that just needs color, not coverage. Besides, heavy make-up on thin skin is aging because it collects in and emphasizes tiny lines. But to get that no–make-up look and still look *terrific*, you can't go it alone . . . you need cosmetics. Here's how to compromise artfully:

℞. *Choose a light, thin foundation*. A whipped soufflé base would be excellent for a woman with skin like Jan's. It is very sheer, so it works well if you just want to even up your skin tone, get a creamy-smooth look, and/or wear very little make-up or like the "unmade-up" look and feel. Because it's so thin, a sheer soufflé also makes great sense if you're not adept with make-up.

℞. *If you're more comfortable with a liquid than a soufflé,* learn how to apply that liquid make-up like a pro. When the liquid is three-quarters dry, study your face and add more where you skipped the first time around. When you make corrections before your make-up is completely dry, you can blend everything into one layer. When you add a dab here and there to already-dry foundation, you run the risk of having a thick, heavy, layered-looking face. When make-up is dry, use your fingertips to blend once more around the nostrils, where liquid may unbecomingly collect.

℞. *Perform scar revision.* Plastic surgeons do it all the time (see Chapter 3), but if you're not ready for the knife, and you have a small scar or dimplelike imperfection that needs softening (look to the side of the mouth in Jan's morning picture), use a camouflage stick at least two shades lighter than your foundation in the "dimple." Dot on 5 or 6 layers to thicken up the indentation. The thick application will fill up the hole a bit; the light color will take away the shadow the indentation creates. Do revision first, apply foundation second. Note how effective this process is in filling out and hiding minor imperfections by studying Jan's unretouched afternoon picture.

℞. *Correct two common eye flaws associated with thin skin.*

Flaw #1: Red-rimmed eyes. I often notice that both the inner and outer lower eyelid of fair, thin-skinned women looks red as these women get older. To fight the red-eyed look, use a cobalt blue pencil specifically designed to line inside the lower lid. Rimming the eye with blue will make the whites of your eyes look whiter.

Flaw #2: Tiny lines on eyelids. If you have generally thin skin, realize the skin around your eyes is thinner yet, and so will tend to develop tiny little lines before the rest of your face. To compensate, wear cream shadow on your upper lids. It won't gather in the lines the way a powder formula might.

To make those little crinkles *under* your eyes look less noticeable, make your own at-home version of the newly popular and expensive "wrinkles off" preparations. Just combine the white of one egg with half as much still mineral water. Brush this mix across undereye area with a small artist's brush and feel skin tighten. Apply make-up base right over it.

℞. *Build up a thin, pursed-looking mouth.* Some women are born thin-lipped; others find their lips look thinner with time. Whatever the case, if you have the problem, the make-up correction involves a lip pencil and the process of "lip building." You *must* use a lip pencil to outline. You cannot build a new border with a tube of lipstick—it's too thick. Many women didn't feel comfortable using the mechanical lead pencil lipliners, but the new all-wood pencils have a softer point, making them easier to wield.

To build a fuller lip, use short strokes and outline one-half of each lip at a time. First, follow the natural contours of your lips so you'll have a base on which to "build," making sure you don't line all the way into the corners of your mouth (which pulls the mouth down).

When your natural lip is outlined, use the same short strokes *just slightly outside* your lipline to get a subtly wider mouth. Feather the line up and out (again *subtle* is the key) at the corners to achieve a happier as well as fuller mouth. You can keep building on additional layers of outline color as long as the result still looks natural. For most attractive results, outline in a darker color, fill in with a softer but vibrant shade in the same family.

℞. *Camouflage a thin-skinned chest (an accompaniment of a thin-skinned face) that allows blue veins and red blood vessels to show through.* If you're thin-skinned all over, your blood vessels may be beginning to peek through. To counteract this problem on your face, a lavender-tinted make-up underbase plus a light, whipped soufflé-type foundation will provide ample coverage. But when you wear a low-cut dress, the problem is also visible on your *chest*.

Of course, you don't want to bring your foundation halfway down your chest—that would be ridiculous. But what you can do is fill a large, long-handled sable make-up brush with your moisturizing powder and dust it a few times over your chest. This will minimize the appearance of veins. It also helps cover any scattered problems the Messy Skin Syndrome may be causing in your chest area without giving your chest a made-up look.

Make-up Postscript

Your lifetime-guarantee make-up buying chart

If you're insecure about make-up and don't have the color-blending skills of a Renaissance "old master," mixing and matching inappropriate cosmetic shades can give you a look that is more garish than glamorous, especially as you pass 30. When you're young and you don't know what you're doing, sea-green eyeshadow, plum lips, and browned cheeks may give you an "interesting" look; the kind-hearted will think you're a free spirit who loves to experiment.

But now that it is more important to avoid coloring errors, it may be gratifying to learn the simple color guidelines that will teach you all you need to know about buying cosmetics—for today and forever.

There are really only two basic make-up options. You will select either the *pink to plum* face (See Column A) or the *honey to mahogany* face

(Column B below), depending on your skin, eye, and hair color.

You're Column A if you have fair skin, *light* brown, blonde, or silver hair, and blue or light green eyes; fair skin, *pale* brown or hazel eyes, and dark hair.

You're Column B if you have olive, ruddy, or sallow skin; very green or dark brown eyes; auburn hair; fair skin, dark eyes, and dark hair.

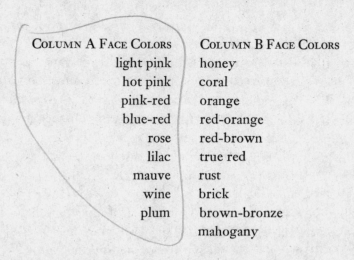

COLUMN A FACE COLORS	COLUMN B FACE COLORS
light pink	honey
hot pink	coral
pink-red	orange
blue-red	red-orange
rose	red-brown
lilac	true red
mauve	rust
wine	brick
plum	brown-bronze
	mahogany

Once you decide which basic palette will complement your face best, you have an almost free hand in choosing which particular shades you will wear. You can move up and down the scale in intensity, keeping just two points in mind:

1. *Fashion.* You certainly don't have to be a slave to a changing cosmetic color wheel, but you will date your looks and age yourself if you don't take current trends into consideration. If you love hot pink, but wines are the color rage, compromise with pink-reds or deeper rose colors, which will still look terrific on you.

Similarly, if you're in the Column B category and it's a true red season but you don't feel comfortable in so violent a color, a slightly muted brick will do the trick.

2. *Your age.* If you're older, you should choose a slightly less intense version of the face of the season. If deep mahogany lips and cheeks are the "now" color, they may look too hard on you. Instead, tone down to the brick or rusts.

The interpretation of the above two options changes from year to year, but if you just juggle the *intensity* to keep in step with fashion and your age, you will look right with the same color palette throughout your whole life.

Adopting a tone-on-tone color scheme will give you a subtle you're-in-control look. Jan, a fair-skinned, dark-eyed brunette, looks good in honeyed/

bronzed tones. A light soufflé foundation in a honey shade covers her thin skin; honey/bronzish cream blusher lights up her cheeks. Her lips are outlined in bronze, filled in with honey. Her eyes feature honey-colored eyeshadow flecked with gold. (Touches of gold will light up anyone's eyes. Manufacturers have muted both the basic shadow colors and the sparkle, so if you look good in brown and bronze, don't wait for evening to warm it up with subtle gold touches.)

Your eye options

You have more leeway with eye color—just make sure the colors you choose don't match (and therefore overpower) your natural eye color.

If you're insecure about make-up, remember that taupe and gray are flattering to all eyes and work equally well with pale pink or deep mahogany cheeks and lips.

Once you become more adept at color coordination you might want to add the following shades:

If you have brown eyes, any deep, smoky colors, including plum, olive, and charcoal, will flatter you.

If you have blue eyes, soft mauves, heathers, and lavenders will work.

If you have green eyes, try navy or metallic-bronze shades.

If you have hazel eyes, pick up warm apricots and toasts as well as gold-flecked colors.

Eye exceptions

Just when you think you have everything all figured out, I have to tell you that if you're over 45, forget the above eye color rules. As you get older, you need brighter colors on your eyes to liven up the slightly faded look that yellowing, red-rimming, and (let's face it) age produce. The taupe and gray that are right for everyone would be too deadly dull as your main eye color, but you can wear them in your eye crease both to hide lines and to keep a high-fashion effect. The smoky olives, plums, and charcoals would also be for your crease only.

But I'm not suggesting you have *carte blanche* to choose any bright shade. If the new colors are "disco fever electric blue" and "wild-eyed emerald green," avoid them. You can find bright, lively eye colors to add a spark of light rather than fright to your face.

Step #4: Body Camouflage

Slim it with clothes

Incorrectly cut clothes, coupled with the wrong undergarments add

10 years and more than 10 pounds to any less-than-trim torso.

The first step is the proper underwear. Good possibilities include a one-piece bra and slip or a body stocking. Don't wear a heavy one-piece bra-girdle combination if you have a few pounds to spare. Heavier women tend to perspire more, and no one wants to look as though she's in a menopausal sweat. Your bra cups should be seamed, and there should be a good separation between them. Seaming adds natural uplift, separation emphasizes cleavage. The whole point: a firm- (which equals young-) looking breast. If you have an ample soft breast and want to wear an uplift bra, make sure there isn't too much overflow. You'll get an unnatural, jiggling effect when the muscles supporting the soft tissue offer little or no support.

To soften anyone's look, what could be softer than silk? Here, a non-clinging silk dress flows loosely over the bust, around the hips and waist. The simple self-fabric belt gives Jan's waist definition, yet it doesn't look as though she's trying to hide anything. The three-quarter sleeve is a graceful length. Compare the A.M. and P.M. arms looks, and you'll see how easily camouflage can hide specific body problems.

Color Cue: Jan looks terrific in turquoise. A bright color is the right color to create a young impression. If the fabric is soft and sensual and the dress glides over your silhouette rather than pulling tightly at each curve, you needn't limit your wardrobe to somber hues.

Step #5: A Little of the Young Razzle-Dazzle

GETTING RID OF THE DAZZLE-ROBBERS

There are certain "good" jewelry fads that come and go, upon which you shouldn't waste your hard-earned dollars (remember "mood" rings, watches, and necklaces a few years back?). There are also jewelry styles that add 10 years to your looks. If you have any of the following that fit into either of the above categories, chalk them up to experience.

These "wastes" include most animal, vegetable or insect pins. The bug perched on Jan's lapel in her morning picture does nothing for her; neither would the run-of-the-mill poodles, owls, daffodils, or other flora and fauna—they all give off an "old" image. Of course, the animal jewelry created by state-of-the-art designers can be works of art. But local Mr. X's interpretation of a dachshund with little beady eyes (even if they *are* rubies) probably should be kept in a kennel. You should also forget ankle bracelets, charm bracelets and necklaces, name or initial jewelry (you know who you are), pieces that noisily announce your entrance before you appear in the room (anything that clangs or rattles—bells are fine for cows, not for you), silver and turquoise jewelry (one piece is fine, but you need not look like the favorite of Geronimo), wearing rings on many fingers, and having your ears pierced with double holes for two sets of earrings (one is enough).

Now take a look at Jan's afternoon jewelry. A delicate thin bracelet cuts the wrist size while a long, simple gold chain with a few small diamonds adds just the right amount of glitter to the neck and throat. A shiny button earring adds sparkle to the face. The gold ring on Jan's pinky shows off long, slender fingers and youthful hands; narrow lapis lazuli bands stacked above and below a wedding band (or any fairly narrow ring) give it a new look. You could also stack with gold rope, enameled or stone-set bands. The possibilities are almost endless if the design is simple.

CHAPTER 20

❦❦❦

Over 55 / Overstatused / Overdone

Step #1: The Strategy

SIMPLIFY IT

In the morning option, Delores and I set out to show how an overdone woman ages herself by submerging her own identity under a jumble of other people's names and initials. When you reach that point in life when you should (or do) have status in your community or crowd, you don't need to proclaim it with a Bill Blass scarf, Dior pocketbook, Oleg Cassini glasscase, Vuitton shopping bag and belt. Delores is a tall, attractive woman who, like so many women, does not need label overkill to look important or expensively pulled together. Our strategy: Take it off, take it all off! Let me show you how to advertise for yourself.

Step #2: Hair Revitalization

SIMPLIFYING AN OVERDONE HAIRSTYLE

In the morning, Delores's hair is so overstyled one also expects it to have been signed by the creator. A too obvious, inexpert attempt to add height and cover a lined forehead produces a wigged effect. This wrong kind of overdone camouflage makes a woman appear dated and harsh looking because all the fullness is in the wrong place. Adding red to her hair produced a shade that's wrong for Delores—not for her age, but for her changing skin tones. The yellow undertones in the red hair pick up the sallowness that many complexions develop as the years pass.

Delores's afternoon cut is easy to maintain and casual looking. A carefree cut is always young. This new styling completely changed the shape of Delores's face by drawing attention to her strong high cheekbones. A little length was left behind the ears to camouflage signs of aging in the back of the neck. Her hair color was softened by adding light brown to replace the red tones and allowing a few golden highlights to peek through. For a closer study of how red hair should look at different ages, see the Time Machine photos and copy, page 259.

Step #3: The 29-and-Holding (Holding, Holding) Corrective Make-up Guide

How to camouflage mature, lined skin

℞. *Hide lots of crisscrossed surface lines and vertical pleating on cheeks* by using more treatment and less make-up. As you get older, more make-up does not cover more, it shows up more flaws because heavier foundations frequently applied tend to collect in tiny facial crevices, outlining them.

First bet: *Soften the crevices* with moisturizing, nourishing treatment products. If you have mature skin, consider the following four pre–make-up steps essential:

1. Nongreasy collagen-containing day cream.

2. Lightweight eye oil (or oil-rich line-softening stick that melts with contact so you don't have to pull delicate skin) that disappears into eye creases, leaving a moist (not thick) look behind.

3. Throat cream (take advantage of its tightening power *at night* by applying under and across your breasts for an extra bit of bosom firming while you sleep).

Intermezzo: Let steps 1 to 3 sink into your skin while you have your morning coffee.

4. Apply moisturizer.

Second bet: Apply a less-is-more lightweight whipped soufflé foundation to even out your skin tone; add a bit of allover color.

Wrong bet: Don't use face powder. Dry, lining skin looks young with a creamy, moist finish. Powder will not only make you look dry, it will also collect in facial lines as the day wears on.

℞. *Cover angular accordion lines running down neck*. Continue your foundation down over your throat. (The only time you need make up your neck is to cover imperfections.)

℞. *For soft-looking, 10-years-younger eyes when the lid is lined*, use only cream shadows or creamy pencils. They won't collect in creases and folds as powders do. What color shadow is best? Brown is the worst for an older woman—it makes a woman of Delores's age and coloring look drab and sad. In Delores's afternoon picture, she wears a subtle greenish blue on the lid near her eye for a bit of color and a candlelight pink across her browbone for a highlight (don't wear pinks flush against your eyeball or you may wind up with a pink-eyed look, which is unattractive if not contagious!).

℞. *To counteract yellowing, watery-looking eyes*, line the inner lower rim of your eyes with cobalt blue (never black if you're over 40) pencil, which will make the "whites" look whiter by comparison.

℞. *To compensate for sparse lashes*, use the smudge eyelining technique. If your eyes have lost some lashes over the years, get the vibrant eye-framing look that lots of mascaraed lash no longer provides by framing your eyes with liner. But just when you need liner, you may find your hands are no longer quite so steady and your vision less than 20/20, both problems that make painting on a flawless liquid line nearly impossible. Years ago, you had no choice. Liquid eyeliner was created for the young beautiful eye *and* the young steady hand.

But now you can outline your eyes by using Q-tips and a soft shadowing pencil made for the eye area (not for brows or lips) that won't pull on soft skin. Draw on 5 dots as close to your upper lid as you can manage (perfection isn't essential). And *smudge* the dots together with a Q-tip (it's like the old connect-the-dots children's game). The result is a *soft* eye-framing line, easily accomplished.

℞. *For a young, moist-looking mouth*, use a pearl-shine lipstick. "Pearlized" *is* an old-fashioned term, but manufacturers put pearl in lipstick for a specific reason: It helps give a shiny, moist-mouth look to older women who can't use gloss because it collects in those tiny vertical lines above the upper lip. Years ago too much pearl created a whitish glow, a problem which long since has been corrected by the industry and changing cosmetic fashion trends; so if you buy your lipstick from a with-it cosmetic company, there will be just enough pearl in the formula to add a *bit* of shine to the muted fashion colors you want. If you wore a flat (no pearl) brown mahogany lip color, it would probably look too dull on you. But with the hint of sparkle the pearl provides, you can have a pinkish-brown, bronzy mouth that's *au courant* and correct.

12 Make-up and Camouflage Ṛs for Women Who Wear Glasses

Ṛ #1. *If you need a strong prescription* but have lots of fine wrinkles on your cheeks, consider a smaller frame. The magnifying effects of your super-strong lenses will not only enable you to read better, they'll enable others to see magnified reproductions of your tiny wrinkles, which are bad enough normal-sized! A smaller-sized frame at least minimizes the area that will be "blown up."

Ṛ #2. *Defy gravity.* If your features seem to be turning downward, don't accentuate the downward "sad" drift by choosing frames so large they seem to droop down onto your cheeks. Droopy eyes and an overhanging upper lid can further be helped by choosing a frame whose upper half slants up and out. If you're developing a bit of a jowl, strong, squared frames will help focus attention on the upper half of your face.

Ṛ #3. *When you try on frames,* wear your everyday eyeshadow and make-up. If you favor rose-colored tinted lenses, you may be surprised to find that the green shadow you usually wear shows up as *mud color* under that slightly pink glass. You'll have to opt for either a different lens color or different eyeshadow.

Ṛ #4. *If you wear large frames,* put on your glasses before your blusher so you're sure your cheek color will be properly placed and visible.

Ṛ #5. *If undereye bags are your nemesis,* wear round frames that are thick rather than thin. Skinny-wired granny glasses won't provide much camouflage.

Ṛ #6. *Compensate for the undereye shadows* that frames cause/accentuate by wearing a lighter color foundation down to where the frames rest. You don't want to use a camouflage stick (which is heavier than foundation) because the lenses will magnify and further thicken your shadow-concealing make-up.

Ṛ #7. *Whatever size frames you choose,* always wear lipstick when wearing glasses. It will help balance your face and keep you from looking like a schoolmarm.

Ṛ #8. *Make sure the top of the frame* rests above your eyebrows or covers them. If your brows show above your glasses, you'll look perpetually surprised.

Ṛ #9. *Don't wear very large dark-colored frames* if you are pale or wear little make-up. Your glasses will overpower your face.

Ṛ #10. *If you have only one pair of glasses,* don't make it a very deep high-fashion color. You will tire of the frames more quickly, they won't go with everything, and the color may go out of style all too quickly.

℞ #11. *If red is your best color* (you always wear red lipstick and red clothes), carry out the theme in your glasses' frames. But rather than get a bright red, consider the subtle color of red-hued Lucite frames. In the same way, purple frames become a subtle lavender tint in Lucite. Subtler hues make a fashion statement without becoming overly important; they work with any outfit.

℞ #12. *If you're older* and the colorful eyeshadows you need are difficult for you to apply, a colorful eyeglass frame will light up your eyes and spark up your face, and there's no tricky application necessary.

Step #4: Body Camouflage

SHED THE LAYERS, CLUTTER, AND INITIALS—
AND SHED 10 YEARS

The bulky, layering effect of scarf, sweater, and jacket makes Delores look bulky and heavy (when she is neither), and her dark, shapeless suit is more than matronly—it's downright aging. Delores has to cover her sweater with a jacket because clingy knits don't really work for large-breasted older women. She needs a seamed bra, but the seams would show through the thin sweater, and there's always the possibility of a bit of midriff bulge or bra overhang being accentuated by a shows-everything little knit. The oversized mock-pearl necklace and earrings make no fashion statement; all they say is big, fake, and pointless.

In the afternoon, we had Delores shed pearls, jacket, scarf, and sweater. She shed all of *their* initials. By shedding the clutter, she also shed 10 years. The real Delores emerges in Option #2, a youthful, secure-looking woman still dressed classically (and classily) but with *simplified* elegance. She wears a flowing V-neck pattern-on-pattern shirt loosely fitted to cover any midriff bulge. The tucks at the shoulders take the emphasis away from a slightly curving back or beginning dowager's hump. From the front, the fleshy parts of a no longer young breast are hidden by fabric; the V is so cut that only the firm part of the chest is visible. Though the belt of the same color is wide, it is soft and crushy; a stiff leather belt of the same width might push the stomach out too far; a soft belt kind of leans into it.

Delores's skirt is sort of a sheath, sort of an A-line; the in-between cut teases fashion to flatter her body. If either straight or very full skirts are "in," and neither looks right on you, go with a skirt that falls loosely around your hips. A classically cut skirt will always look right, while a classic fabric—a thin light wool or summer linen—says you know quality (though you have to be careful: linen creases so easily I'd never wear it on a plane). It's always better to invest in good fabrics than in fancy name labels.

What about undergarments? Even if fashion says go naked except for laced-up sandals, most older women do need firming. The body stocking and nonpaneled slimmer are good choices, depending on your needs. But skip the all-paneled, hooked and zippered harness even if it narrows you a bit more. In the process, the harness/girdle will cause you to have that stiff, can't-move-or-breathe look that hasn't been associated with youth since Scarlett strutted around Tara.

Step #5: A Little of the Young Razzle-Dazzle

DIAMONDS ARE FOREVER

You needn't flash a "piece of the rock" that would make the men at De Beers blink to get the classy glitter that only diamonds can provide. In fact, because understated jewelry is always right, not being able to afford a 7-carat blinder may add rather than detract from your well-dressed packaging. I have many wealthy clients who go out of their way to avoid the one-giant-stone look, and one of the ways they go is with *pavé* diamonds, many small stones the same size set flush with the surface and very close together to give the look of lots of *subtle* sparkle.

Delores is wearing one good piece of jewelry in the form of a *pavé* diamond necklace, and the look is elegant and ageless against her good throat.

You may have the makings of a *pavé*-look piece tucked away in your jewelry box. If you're divorced and have a small-stoned diamond wedding band you no longer wear, if you have grandmother's cocktail ring that misses the deco period and no longer suits your fancy, or if you have several small diamonds from assorted jewelry you no longer wear (old pinky or signet rings, old-fashioned charm bracelets, pins or earrings), you can have them reset together into one important piece. Remember, fine jewelers are also designers, and with the price of diamonds recently rising, you should consider restyling rather than investing in new stones. Many stones set close together (even if the stones are not all the same size) can give a contemporary new-jewelry look and help you turn dust-gatherers into important fashion pieces.

Here, some diamond facts from Finlay: Diamond weight is measured in carats (with a *c*, as opposed to the *k* used to measure gold karats). No matter where in the world you buy them, 1 ounce equals 142 carats; 1 carat equals 100 points. If you're looking at small stones, you'll talk to the jeweler about points. If you're looking at a stone of 1 carat or more (let's say for a pendant, earring, or engagement ring), you should know something about how quality is judged.

There are four determinants of diamond value: carat, clarity, color, and cut. *Carat* refers to the weight (size) of the stone; *clarity* deals with imperfections or flaws within or upon the surface that interfere with the passage of light through that stone. External flaws are called blemishes; internal defects are called inclusions.

Flawless stones of fine quality are very expensive today, but there is nothing wrong with buying and wearing slightly flawed stones of less than perfect color. Frequently, imperfections are not noticeable to the naked eye and such stones are priced very much better than absolutely perfect diamonds.

Perfect *cut* means the diamond in question has been cut to ideal proportions and is well finished.

Color. Highly transparent, colorless diamonds are the most valuable. Equally pricey are rare colors: pink, blue, green, violet, canary, or strong brown (pale yellow and pale brown are not rare, and so are not as valuable as clear stones).

One important point: Unless you have more than one piece, you don't want to save your diamonds for special occasions. Have the stones designed and set in a simple style that will allow you to wear them frequently. I'm not suggesting you bejewel yourself to play tennis—but you should be able to wear simple diamond jewelry to work or for any daytime (as well as evening) occasion.

One important bonus: Diamonds are the hardest mineral known to man, so you don't have to worry about denting, scratching, or chipping with most normal use.

CHAPTER 21

❦❦❦

The Hair Color Time Machine:
How to Change Your Hair Color
As Time Changes You

Hair color can do marvelous things for a woman at any age. But the same shades that add drama and glamour to a 25-year-old may look too flashy on a 35-year-old, and downright harsh framing a 45-plus face. You *do* have to consider those first lines when covering first grays.

As part of my Fail-Proof Hair Tint Selection System, I want you to study the Time Machine photos in the color insert. I have taken three of our *What a Difference a Day Makes* candidates and (through the magic of re-touching) shown you how their faces might look if they were 10 years older or younger than their present age. Master hair colorists Terry Foster and Le-land Hirsch (the latter is responsible for the plum/aubergine/wine high-lights in my own hair . . . and also lends his expertise to the beauty pages of top fashion magazines) suggested the hair colors that would work best for the changing faces of in-between women. If you see yourself in one of these photos, here's what you should know.

BLONDES

Age 25-Plus: Platinum Blonde Bombshell

If you want to be platinum, do it now, before it's too late! The pre-requisites are clear, unblemished, and unlined skin (not to mention the delicate pale coloring and blue eyes that Rose comes by naturally), which you'll highlight with pink to plum make-up. If you go platinum when you're much older, you run the risk of being mistaken for a Mae West impersonator. As shown in Rose's picture, you should have your eyebrows lightened to a smoky platinum shade. No one will really believe you're a *natural* platinum (not if you're over the age of 12), but why let too-dark brows destroy a beautiful illusion?

Age 35-Plus: Sunny Honey Blonde

Consider this rule of thumb: As you add a year, add a toner just one shade darker. Rose's actual unretouched photo, showing the way she looks today, is proof that subtle honey color with more depth and richness best complements 35-year-old skin. Light honey-brown brows and red lipstick complete the look.

Age 45-Plus: Blonde Brown

When you reach this plateau, your thin skin may start to crumple and wrinkle (just like thin tissue paper). You will need a softer blonde frame, but you still want to retain the brightness of youth. Try tinting the hair a dark blonde, then highlighting a few selected strands at a time using the foil method explained in Part Five. The result: Golden highlights without that tried-too-hard, brassy look.

BRUNETTES

Age 25-Plus: Sultry Brunette

Margarita's natural brown-black hair shows that Nature knows what she's doing when picking hair color to complement a young face. If you're olive-skinned, you can wear almost black hair colors now. If your dark hair is not as rich looking as Margarita's, consider intensifying the shade with henna.

Age 35-Plus: Warm Brown

When you reach 35 and you are olive- rather than fair- and thin-skinned, your complexion changes may not be markedly different from your mid-to-late-20s look (your nose-to-mouth lines may deepen a bit; perhaps your forehead and undereye areas are not quite as smooth as they used to be). Your subtly changing skin will look best against subtly lightened hair. A warm brown glow should replace your black-brown hair.

Age 45-Plus: Chestnut Brown

Look at Margarita's first picture and the 45-plus version. You'll see the hair is lightened quite a bit to soften the look of a woman who now has definite lines on her face and throat. (Remember, very dark hair makes wrinkles seem even more prominent.) A medium chestnut shade is further highlighted with subtle five-hairs-at-a-time streaking (only a colorist can do this) in a lighter brown. This brown-on-brown golden/chestnut look is especially effective on formerly dark brown hair that is now shot through with gray.

REDHEADS

Age 35-Plus: Strawberry Red

You can see from Delores's current age (55-plus) photo that she still has beautiful skin, so I don't think I'm too far off the mark in assuming that her 35-year-old face was very clear and unlined. If you're 35-plus and still have clear, beautiful English-type skin (and green eyes), you can still be a dramatically glamorous shade of red (if you were going blonde, and had all of the above assets, it would already be time to tone down a bit). Just make sure to combine vibrant hair color with soft make-up and a soft-looking hairstyle as we have done here. Notice Delores is wearing a muted cinder green eyeshadow; bright green would be aging.

If you're in this age bracket and you want to go red, yet you have a more olive skin tone and brown eyes, as I do, consider my color choice: the plum/wine reds, also called aubergine. (Note from Leland: Don't confuse aubergine/wine/plum tones with auburn hair colorings. Auburn is brown mixed with orange dyes, and aubergine is brown with red dyes. Many women mistakenly ask for auburn when they really want aubergine, and vice versa.) No matter how red/plum your hair, you need a muted (never fire-engine) shade on your brows; your colorist will be able to mix the proper subtle brow shade.

Age 45-Plus: Apricot Red

Lines on the face signal the need for less obvious hair color. Here, a softer, more apricot shade (the result of brown tones blended into the red) offers a light frame for the face and blends well with gray. The more unusual strawberry shades should be left behind at this point.

Age 55-Plus: Light Brown Warmed with Copper

Today Delores wears the softest of the soft; there should be no hint of fire-engine hues in over-50 hair. Golden copper highlights give a lift to light brown hair. The color here is bright enough to give a lift to an older woman's face, but there is nothing harsh about it.

EPILOGUE

✿✿✿

Now that you've completed your study of my subtract-10-years system, I'd like to share with you the last lines of a poem sent me by a "friend" of an early reader of this manuscript.

Dammit, she has to be 40 if she's a day.
Only formaldehyde, Lucifer, or
Adrien Arpel could have preserved her
that way.

Index

❧❧❧

Here are two more Warner books to help you look and feel better:

THE 15-MINUTE-A-DAY *NATURAL* FACE LIFT

Now you can give yourself all the beautifying effects of a face lift—safely and naturally without surgery—through a unique series of exercises created by international beauty expert M.J. Saffon. In just minutes a day you can:

Smooth the forehead

Banish frowns

Round out hollow cheeks

Prevent or firm puffy eyelids

Strengthen, smooth and tone the entire eye area

Erase crow's feet

Shape the lips

Erase lines around the mouth

Tighten and smooth neck muscles

Remove a double chin

Firm the entire face

A large format quality paperback

L97788-8 $3.95 (U.S.A.)
L97849-3 $4.95 (Canada)

NEVER-SAY-DIET BOOK

Richard Simmons has a new idea for helping you take weight off slowly and safely so that you can keep it off forever—without drugs, pills, or dangerous diuretics, without the hassles of calorie counters, lists of forbidden foods, or boring daily menus.

You may know Simmons from *General Hospital,* the top-rated day-time drama, where he appears as himself, owner of the famous exercise studio in Beverly Hills. His studio has helped such people as Dustin Hoffman, Barbra Streisand, Henry Winkler, and Diana Ross.

Join the thousands of people who have found the key to success with Simmons' important body-correcting program, including thirty-two exercises to correct problem areas from bags under the eyes to fat thighs, buttocks, stomach, and arms.

Available in hardcover
L51209-5 $14.95

Look for these—and other Warner best-sellers—in your bookstore. If you can't find them, you may order directly from us by sending your check or money order for the retail price of the book plus 50¢ per order and 50¢ per copy to cover postage and handling to: WARNER BOOKS, P.O. Box 690, New York, NY 10019. N.Y. State and California residents must add applicable sales tax. Please allow 4 weeks for delivery of your books.